# Cardiovascular Assessment of the Adult Patient

*Commissioning Editor:* Rita Demetriou-Swanwick
*Development Editors:* Veronika Watkins/Clive Hewat
*Project Manager:* Anita Somaroutu
*Designer/Design Direction:* Charles Gray
*Illustration Manager:* Merlyn Harvey
*Illustrator:* Robert Britton

# Cardiorespiratory Assessment of the Adult Patient
## A Clinician's Guide

*Edited by*

### Mary-Ann Broad BSc, MSc, MCSP
*Clinical Specialist Physiotherapist,
Cardiff and Vale University Health Board, Cardiff, UK*

### Matthew Quint Grad Dip Phys, MPhil, MCSP
*Respiratory Clinical Specialist,
Solent Primary Care NHS Trust, Portsmouth, UK*

### Sandy Thomas M Ed, Cert Ed, Dip TP, MCSP
*Senior Lecturer, University of the West of England,
Bristol, UK*

### Paul Twose BSc, MCSP
*Specialist Band 6 Physiotherapist,
Cardiff and Vale University Health Board, Cardiff, UK*

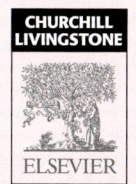

CHURCHILL LIVINGSTONE
ELSEVIER

Edinburgh   London   New York   Oxford   Philadelphia
St Louis   Sydney   Toronto   2012

# CHURCHILL LIVINGSTONE
ELSEVIER

© 2012 Elsevier Ltd. All rights reserved.

No part of this publication may be reproduced or transmitted in any form or by any means, electronic or mechanical, including photocopying, recording, or any information storage and retrieval system, without permission in writing from the publisher. Details on how to seek permission, further information about the Publisher's permissions policies and our arrangements with organizations such as the Copyright Clearance Center and the Copyright Licensing Agency, can be found at our website: www.elsevier.com/permissions.

This book and the individual contributions contained in it are protected under copyright by the Publisher (other than as may be noted herein).

ISBN: 978 0 7020 4345 1

**British Library Cataloguing in Publication Data**
A catalogue record for this book is available from the British Library

**Library of Congress Cataloging in Publication Data**
A catalog record for this book is available from the Library of Congress

**Notices**
Knowledge and best practice in this field are constantly changing. As new research and experience broaden our understanding, changes in research methods, professional practices, or medical treatment may become necessary.

Practitioners and researchers must always rely on their own experience and knowledge in evaluating and using any information, methods, compounds, or experiments described herein. In using such information or methods they should be mindful of their own safety and the safety of others, including parties for whom they have a professional responsibility.

With respect to any drug or pharmaceutical products identified, readers are advised to check the most current information provided (i) on procedures featured or (ii) by the manufacturer of each product to be administered, to verify the recommended dose or formula, the method and duration of administration, and contraindications. It is the responsibility of practitioners, relying on their own experience and knowledge of their patients, to make diagnoses, to determine dosages and the best treatment for each individual patient, and to take all appropriate safety precautions.

To the fullest extent of the law, neither the Publisher nor the authors, contributors, or editors, assume any liability for any injury and/or damage to persons or property as a matter of products liability, negligence or otherwise, or from any use or operation of any methods, products, instructions, or ideas contained in the material herein.

ELSEVIER
your source for books, journals and multimedia in the health sciences
www.elsevierhealth.com

Working together to grow libraries in developing countries
www.elsevier.com | www.bookaid.org | www.sabre.org
ELSEVIER  BOOK AID International  Sabre Foundation

The Publisher's policy is to use paper manufactured from sustainable forests

Printed in China

# Contents

**Preface** vii

**How to use this book** ix

**1 An introduction to cardiorespiratory physiotherapy: respiratory assessment**   1

**2 Assessment checklists**   9

**3 Assessment tools**   23

**4 Case scenarios**   173

**Index**   187

# Preface

This book aims to give physiotherapy students and those new to respiratory care a simple, easy-to-use guide to the process and procedures used in the assessment of adult respiratory patients.

Chapter 1 identifies the scope of respiratory physiotherapy. It lists some key aims of physiotherapy assessment and gives an overview of different assessment approaches. It also presents some of the particular issues facing the community respiratory physiotherapist.

Chapter 2 provides a selection of 'assessment checklists' for the main clinical settings that the physiotherapist is likely to encounter. These can be used as an *'aide-memoire'* to help ensure that each patient assessment includes everything relevant. Although there may appear to be a lot of similarity between these checklists, in practice the approach and prioritization are likely to be very different, depending on the setting and the type of patient. Key points have therefore been included to help students to prioritize and identify what to focus on and prioritize in each setting.

Chapter 3 is an alphabetical selection of 'assessment tools', including those that physiotherapists may be expected to carry out themselves and those where we only need to be able to interpret the assessment findings. These tools include a step-by-step guide to the procedure involved (where relevant), and an explanation of the key findings and their significance for the physiotherapist.

# How to use this book

Read the introduction to respiratory assessment (Chapter 1) and then select the appropriate assessment checklists from Chapter 2 for the setting you are working in and use these as a guide to the assessment process. You may find it useful to discuss the checklist with your supervisor and add any specific assessment procedures that may be used in your particular clinical environment.

Identify from the checklist the procedures you will need to use (or analyse) and then locate these alphabetically within the assessment tools section. Follow the step-by-step guidelines provided.

## PATIENT CONSENT

*Consent is a must!* The patient has to give their consent prior to you commencing any procedure. This needs to be documented, in terms of what they have or have not consented to, how they gave consent (verbally) and what they have not consented to, e.g. 'I do not want to be suctioned'. Remember the Mental Capacity Act and assume that the patient is able to make the decision unless there is evidence otherwise. It is also the patient's right to make a decision you disagree with. For further details on consent, see 3.18 Consent in this text and Harden et al (2009), Chapter 2; see Further Reading.

## INFECTION CONTROL

It is too easy to forget infection control, especially when under pressure, but these principles are there to *protect you and the patient*. These risks are real and there are documented cases of therapists being infected by patients with dangerous diseases (such as pulmonary TB) or passing on infections to patients. It is essential to take precautions in order to limit the spread of infection in any setting (e.g. effective hand washing, cleansing of equipment, use of masks or protective clothing and protective gloves where appropriate).

## DOCUMENTATION

All documentation should be completed in a timely manner, ideally as soon as possible after seeing the patient, and should follow the current Chartered Society of Physiotherapy guidelines (see Further Reading). Ensure that all your documentation is clear and legible. Date and sign each new entry (you may also need to include the time). You should include clear SMART goals, i.e. *S*pecific, *M*easurable, *A*chievable, *R*ealistic and *T*imed. It takes time to learn how to do this – your supervisor will assist you. Discussing the issues with your patient will help you both reach a common consensus and may have an impact on what they agree to do!

## ABBREVIATIONS

The assessment checklists have used abbreviations throughout to keep them concise. These abbreviations are defined in full at first mention within the assessment tools section, and commonly used abbreviations have been included in the pull-out section together with some common normal values.

## FURTHER READING

Chartered Society of Physiotherapy, 2000. *General Principles of Record Keeping and Access to Health Records.* Chartered Society of Physiotherapy, London, UK. Available at: http://www.csp.org.uk/director/members/libraryandpublications/csppublications.cfm?item_id=74C8733B9EF7296ADB1798E7C4F1CFEA

Harden, B., Cross, J., Broad, M., et al, 2009. *Respiratory Physiotherapy: An On-call Survival Guide*, 2nd edn. Churchill Livingstone, Edinburgh, UK.

# CHAPTER 1

# An introduction to cardiorespiratory physiotherapy: respiratory assessment

1.1 The Scope of Respiratory Physiotherapy  1
1.2 Why do We Assess?  4
1.3 Aims of Respiratory Assessment  4
1.4 Assessment Approaches  5
1.5 Assessment in the Community  5
1.6 Clinical Reasoning in Respiratory Care  7

## 1.1 THE SCOPE OF RESPIRATORY PHYSIOTHERAPY

Patients with respiratory problems are encountered in many different settings, from long-term care in the community to critically ill patients on an intensive therapy unit (ITU) (also known as critical care) (Figs 1.1–1.3). Respiratory care may be an integral part of the patient's management in secondary care (hospital) settings, such as respiratory, medical, and surgical and orthopaedic wards as well as burns, care of the elderly, paediatric, neurological, neurosurgical and oncology units. It may also be required for patients with mental health problems or learning disabilities. Physiotherapists work in many of these settings and also within primary care (in the community) for the longer-term rehabilitation of these patients. They may be employed in multiprofessional 'rapid response' or 'early discharge' teams, in which they share the responsibility for assessing and managing acutely ill patients in their own home.

This book will cover physiotherapy assessment in any of the above settings. It is recognized that our role with many respiratory patients may be directed more towards function and rehabilitation than towards specific respiratory problems. Although the focus of this book will be on the assessment of the cardiovascular and respiratory systems, the checklists and tools also include reference to some generic assessment procedures (e.g. functional assessment)

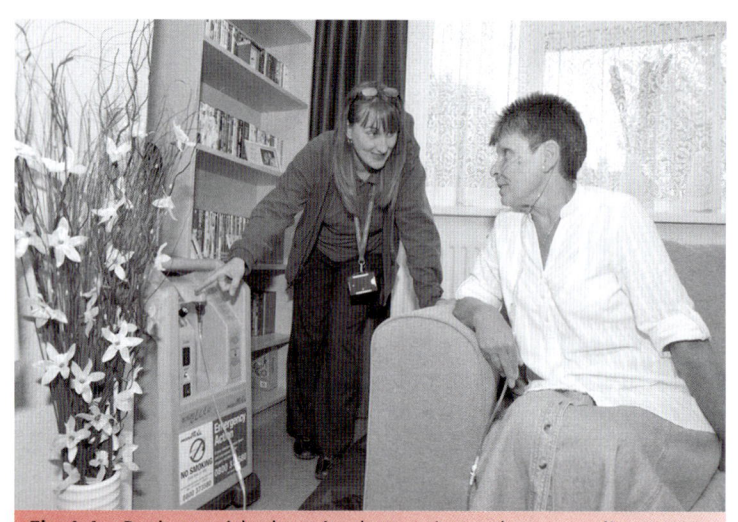

**Fig 1.1** Patient with chronic obstructive pulmonary disease at home with oxygen.

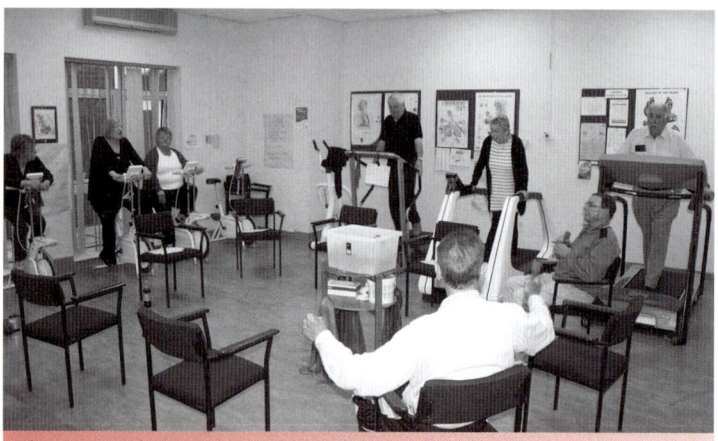

**Fig 1.2** Pulmonary rehabilitation.

and aspects of musculoskeletal and neurological assessment (e.g. pain assessment and muscle testing); however, these have not been considered in detail and the reader is directed to other books in the toolkit series for further information.

The case history in Box 1.1 illustrates the scope of respiratory physiotherapy.

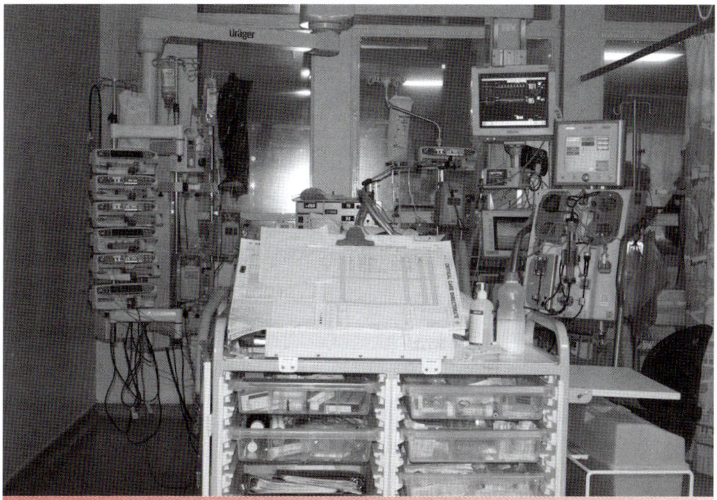

## 1.1 The scope of respiratory physiotherapy

**Fig 1.3** The intensive therapy unit (critical care) setting.

### Box 1.1

Bob Fleming is a 68 year old man with chronic obstructive pulmonary disease who presented to his GP with a chronic productive cough and shortness of breath; he was referred to an outpatient physiotherapist, who taught him some strategies for airway clearance.

At this point, it was noted that he had slowly declining exercise tolerance, and so was referred on to the community pulmonary rehabilitation team. This improved his exercise tolerance, reduced his breathlessness and he was delighted.

Two years later he had his first significant exacerbation of his disease, and was admitted to hospital via the emergency department. He developed type II respiratory failure and was commenced on non-invasive ventilation and transferred to a critical care unit. The medical ward physiotherapist assisted in the setting up and monitoring of his non-invasive ventilation.

Although, initially, he improved, later that day he deteriorated to the point where he required intubation and invasive ventilation. His respiratory status and early rehabilitation were managed by the critical care physiotherapist.

From critical care he was discharged to a respiratory ward, where his therapy continued. He was given an early discharge, requiring regular observation and review; therefore, he was placed in the care of the early discharge team, which included a physiotherapist.

Once stable, he was referred back to the pulmonary rehabilitation team in order to help him return to his preadmission level of ability.

## 1.2 WHY DO WE ASSESS?

When assessing a patient you should have a clear idea of the purpose of the assessment before you start. There may be several aims of a 'respiratory' assessment (see 1.3 Aims of respiratory assessment); although all or most of these issues may need to be addressed at some point, it is necessary to prioritize which are the most significant at the time of assessment. Be aware that priorities may change, and you need to be flexible and responsive to changes in the patient's condition and situation.

## 1.3 AIMS OF RESPIRATORY ASSESSMENT

Assessment may be carried out in order to:

- identify patients requiring immediate CPR (cardiopulmonary resuscitation) – patient safety!
- identify the need for respiratory support – such as oxygen therapy or ventilation
- identify patients requiring specific physiotherapy treatment for sputum retention, loss of volume or breathlessness
- select appropriate physiotherapy management options for managing sputum retention, loss of volume or breathlessness
- identify patients who need to be referred to the medical team for review, such as those who do not appear to be on optimum medication (e.g. steroids or bronchodilators) or those who require further investigations (e.g. chest X-rays or lung function tests)
- determine whether patients can be safely managed at home or whether they need to be in hospital (discharge planning for those in hospital, or admission decisions for patients at home)
- identify any support (e.g. social or medical) the patient may require in order to be discharged from hospital or remain at home
- identify and rate the patient's functional ability and level of independence in activities of daily living
- identify the patient's goals, e.g. in relation to improving mobility, function or social participation
- select appropriate physiotherapy management options for enabling functional ability and independence, and make referrals to other multidisciplinary team members
- facilitate the prescription of an exercise programme that is appropriate for the patient's physical, psychological and social situation
- assess a patient's suitability for pulmonary or cardiac rehabilitation
- assess a patient before and/or after intervention as an outcome measure for audit or research.

The assessment procedures that you use and the significance of the assessment findings will vary according to the patient's situation and the stage in the patient's pathway of care.

## 1.4 ASSESSMENT APPROACHES

Physiotherapy assessment of the respiratory patient may be classified into three main approaches:

- systems-based assessment
- functional assessment
- goal-oriented assessment.

### *SYSTEMS-BASED ASSESSMENT*

A systematic and comprehensive protocol that assesses each body system in turn, following a specified format based on the medical model used by doctors. It focuses on body structure and function and is mainly used in hospital and acute community settings.

### *FUNCTIONAL ASSESSMENT*

This focuses on functional independence and mobility for patients with impairment due to breathlessness, the elderly and those with co-morbidities. It is often used in community settings and with hospital patients prior to discharge.

### *GOAL-ORIENTED ASSESSMENT*

This type of assessment combines aspects of systems-based and functional assessment but with a particular focus on goal setting in order to provide a patient-centred approach. This requires a flexible, tailored assessment that is likely to differ for each patient and does not fit into a prescribed protocol.

These three approaches represent the three domains of 'body structure and function', 'activity' and 'participation' that have been identified in the International Classification of Functioning, Disability and Health, produced by the World Health Organization (see Further reading) (Fig. 1.4).

## 1.5 ASSESSMENT IN THE COMMUNITY

When visiting patients in their own home, assessment priorities may vary depending on whether you are working with acutely ill patients (e.g. in a 'hospital at home' or 'early discharge' team)

# 6 AN INTRODUCTION TO CARDIORESPIRATORY PHYSIOTHERAPY

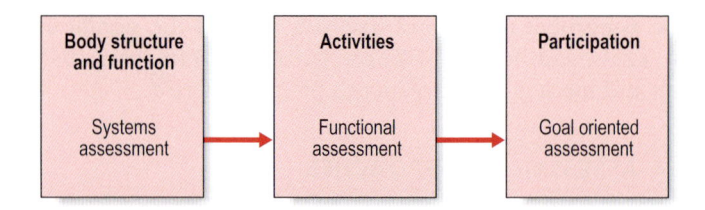

**Fig 1.4** Physiotherapy assessment follows a biopsychosocial approach. All three components of assessment are used at some stage, but the degree of contribution may change from patient to patient.

or whether you are visiting patients who are medically stable for rehabilitation purposes.

With an acutely ill patient, your role may involve making a decision about whether the patient needs admission to hospital or whether he or she requires urgent medical care in order to remain at home (Fig. 1.5). With more stable patients, your priority may be towards optimizing their mobility, function and quality of life to help them to achieve their personal goals and optimum potential. Assessment of an acute respiratory patient in the community setting requires analysis of medical, functional, environmental and social situations, which may be liable to change.

Clinical reasoning therefore requires ongoing re-evaluation of the risk of managing the patient at home, and any decision to admit the patient to hospital is made in accordance with national guidelines (e.g. those produced by the National Institute for Health and Clinical Excellence 2010; see Further reading) and also taking into account the local health and social provision. Some criteria are clear (e.g. unconscious or acutely confused patient), but many are dependent on local services and skills of staff. Patients have the right to choose where treatment is delivered. Discuss all treatment options and risks with patients so that a joint decision can be made, and liaise with other members of the multidisciplinary team.

> *Top tip!*
> Assessment in the community is not fixed and you need to be able to adapt to a situation that changes quickly – do not be afraid to ask for help as this can be challenging.

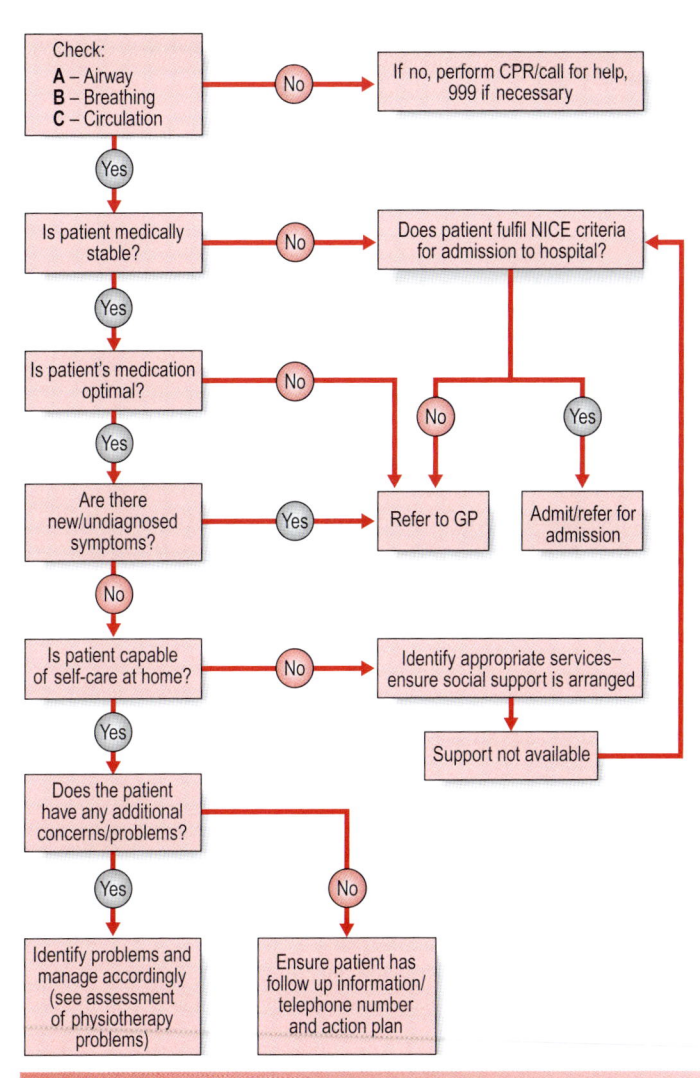

**Fig 1.5** Acute patient in the community decision-making flowchart.

CPR, cardiopulmonary resuscitation; NICE, National Institute for Health and Clinical Excellence.

## 1.6 CLINICAL REASONING IN RESPIRATORY CARE

Cardiorespiratory assessment is not just about being able to perform the assessment techniques. The implications of the results must be considered and links to other findings and the clinical picture must be made.

At the end of your assessment you should ask yourself:

- What problems does the patient have?
- Is the patient likely to respond to physiotherapy?

Problems related to respiration are frequently classified as one or more of the following:

- sputum retention
- volume loss
- increased work of breathing (breathlessness)
- respiratory failure.

The patient's problems may be more generic, such as pain, anxiety, reduced exercise tolerance, functional and mobility limitations, or social problems. Once these problems have been identified, the clinical reasoning process proceeds to treatment planning and implementation, which are not in the remit of this book. Readers may find *Respiratory Physiotherapy: An On-call Survival Guide* (Harden et al 2009; see Further reading) helpful with regard to managing the respiratory problems listed above.

### FURTHER READING

Harden, B., Cross, J., Broad, M., et al, 2009. Respiratory Physiotherapy: An On-call Survival Guide, 2nd edn. Churchill Livingstone, Edinburgh, UK.

National Institute for Health and Clinical Excellence, 2010. Management of Chronic Obstructive Pulmonary Disease in Adults in Primary and Secondary Care. Clinical Guideline 12. NICE, London, UK. Available at: http://www.nice.org.uk/nicemedia/live/13029/49399/49399.pdf/

World Health Organization, 2011. International Classification of Functioning, Disability and Health. WHO, Geneva, Switzerland. Available at: http://www.who.int/classifications/icf/en/

# CHAPTER 2

# Assessment checklists

2.1 General Assessment  9
2.2 Acute Respiratory Assessment  9
2.3 Rehabilitation Assessment  12
2.4 General Surgery Patients  12
2.5 Critical Care/ITU Patients  13
2.6 Medical Patients  15
2.7 Goal-Oriented Assessment  16
2.8 Functional Assessment  17
2.9 Acute Community Patient Assessment  19

This chapter provides step-by-step checklists, guiding those with little experience of respiratory assessment through the process. Experienced clinicians rarely follow a checklist rigidly. They are quickly able to prioritize, and may deviate from, or expand on, particular aspects when appropriate. In order to develop this skill, you need to be aware of the purpose of each assessment element and relate this to the overall aim(s) of your assessment.

## 2.1 GENERAL ASSESSMENT

An overview of a general assessment is suggested in Tables 2.1 and 2.2.

In any setting, your initial observation of the patient is key, as this will allow you to identify a situation that may require immediate action.

## 2.2 ACUTE RESPIRATORY ASSESSMENT

Use the systems-based checklist (Table 2.3). Your main aim is to decide whether the patient has physiotherapy-related problems (such as sputum retention, volume loss, breathlessness or

### Table 2.1 General assessment: part 1

| **General observations** | |
|---|---|
| If the patient looks well, and is reading the paper – they probably are well! You still need to make sure you do not miss any significant issues | • Face: colour, expression<br>• Condition: clean and well groomed or neglected and unkempt?<br>• Position: in bed, chair or ambulant?<br>• Posture: slumped or upright? Still or restless?<br>• Weight: overweight or underweight, emaciated?<br>• Attachments: note presence of drips, drains and equipment<br>• Skin: wounds, pressure areas, colour, temperature<br>• Peripheries: clubbing, swelling/oedema, cyanosis |
| **ABC** | |
| A quick check from the end of the bed can be crucial in establishing the stability of the patient<br>Always make sure that the patient is not in any immediate danger by assessing their Airway, Breathing and Circulation, and implementing basic life support if required | • *Airway:* is it patent and protected? If not, call for help and establish an airway<br>• *Breathing:* is the patient ventilating efficiently? If not, call for help and support ventilation<br>• *Circulation:* does the patient have an adequate cardiac output? If not, call for help and support circulation |
| Can you recognize these signs and do you know how to address them? If not, you need an update on basic life support | |

### Table 2.2 General assessment: part 2

| For all assessments, it is assumed that informed consent (as appropriate) is sought and documented | |
|---|---|
| **Database**<br>Compile initial database of key information from relevant sources, e.g. medical notes, nursing records, other staff, the patient, carers or relatives as appropriate | • PC<br>• HPC<br>• PMH<br>• DH<br>• SH |
| **Subjective questions** | • How patient is feeling today<br>• Emotional status<br>• Symptoms and pain<br>• Fatigue<br>• Specific problems |

PC, presenting complaint or condition; HPC, history of present condition; PMH, past medical history; DH, drug history; SH, social history.

## 2.2 Acute respiratory assessment

**Table 2.3 Systems-based assessment outline**

| | |
|---|---|
| Central nervous system (CNS) | • Level of consciousness (may use AVPU or GCS)<br>• Sedation score<br>• Pupils: size and reactivity<br>• ICP<br>• CPP<br>• External ventricular drain (EVD)<br>• Pain score and route of analgesia |
| Cardiovascular system (CVS) | • HR and rhythm<br>• BP and MAP<br>• CVP<br>• Temperature<br>• Invasive cardiac monitoring<br>• Blood (haematology) results as appropriate |
| Renal system (Renal) | • Fluid output, including NG, drains, UO<br>• Fluid input: note the name of all infusions and be aware of what they do as they may affect your treatment options<br>• Renal results as appropriate |
| Respiratory system (RS) | • Mode of ventilation and method of delivery, e.g. ETT, tracheostomy, FM<br>• Ventilator settings<br>• Oxygen delivered: mode of delivery and use of home oxygen<br>• Oxygen saturations, pulse oximetry<br>• Respiratory rate<br>• ABGs<br>• CXR<br>• Pulmonary function tests<br>• Auscultation<br>• Palpation<br>• Percussion note<br>• Cough<br>• Sputum<br>• Breathlessness<br>• Cyanosis<br>• Work and pattern of breathing<br>• Chest wall shape and expansion |

**12** ASSESSMENT CHECKLISTS

| Musculoskeletal system (MS) | • Exercise tolerance<br>• Exercise test such as the 6 minute walk test<br>• Use of aids<br>• Limitations secondary to other injuries, external fixators or plaster casts<br>• Muscle charting/grading |

ABG, arterial blood gas; AVPU, Awake, Voice, Pain, Unrouseable; BP, blood pressure; CPP, cerebral perfusion pressure; CVP, central venous pressure; CXR, chest radiograph; ETT, endotracheal tube; FM, face mask; GCS, Glasgow Coma Scale; HR, heart rate; ICP, intracranial pressure; MAP, mean arterial pressure; NG, nasogastric; UO, urine output.

respiratory failure). You also need to determine whether the patient's condition is stable enough for your selected physiotherapy treatments. The other main purpose of assessment is to identify any deterioration in the patient's condition and ensure that appropriate actions are taken by the healthcare team.

The checklist assumes that the general assessment (Tables 2.1 and 2.2) has already been followed. Specific adaptations for patients in general surgery, critical care and medical settings are then provided (Tables 2.4–2.6). Depending on the setting, different elements may need to be included or omitted (e.g. pupil size may not be monitored regularly in a rehabilitation setting but may be more important in a critical care/intensive therapy unit (ITU) or surgery setting).

## 2.3 REHABILITATION ASSESSMENT

Once decisions about the patient's immediate management have been made, use the goal-oriented and functional checklists, which focus on helping patients achieve their potential or returning them to the status they were at before they deteriorated. You must continue to ensure that your patient remains medically stable, however, and so you may still need to incorporate aspects of the systems approach. A specific checklist for acute patients in the community is also provided (see Table 2.11).

## 2.4 GENERAL SURGERY PATIENTS (Table 2.4)

- Assessment should be specific to the type of surgery.
- Initial assessment focuses on the identification of high-risk patients, according to the likelihood that they could develop cardiorespiratory or mobility complications postoperatively.

## 2.5 Critical care/ITU patients

| Table 2.4 | General surgery: specific considerations |
|---|---|
| Database | • Note the history leading up to surgery and whether elective or emergency admission<br>• Operation notes should be documented, including:<br>– Name of surgery<br>– Incision site<br>– Findings and procedure<br>– Surgery time<br>– Postoperative instructions |
| CNS | • Adequate pain control is key to the optimal management of the surgical patient and must be assessed (see 3.45 Pain scoring) |
| CVS | • Haemoglobin levels, WCC, lactate and CRP are particularly useful for indicating postoperative complications, such as circulatory failure and infection (see 3.6 Blood results) |
| Renal | • Use fluid balance to help identify patients at risk of shock<br>• Note dehydration, which could cause viscous secretions (see 3.58 Sputum assessment)<br>• Note the name of all infusions and be aware of what they do as they may have an impact on your treatment options |
| RS | • Focus on breathing pattern (especially expansion) and cough effectiveness to identify any respiratory complications associated with loss of volume, sputum retention or respiratory failure |
| MS | • Identify any PMH that might lead to functional limitations. Assess function prior to discharge as relevant, e.g. stair assessment, social work review |

CRP, C-reactive protein; PMH, past medical history; WCC, white cell count.

Risk factors commonly considered include age, weight (body mass index), smoking, respiratory disease, upper abdominal incision and length of surgery. In some hospitals, low-risk patients are not routinely reviewed by a physiotherapist.
- Patients should be considered holistically, as reduced levels of mobility can have an impact on discharge planning.

## 2.5 CRITICAL CARE/ITU PATIENTS (Table 2.5)

- Critical care is often considered a daunting environment to those new to cardiorespiratory care. There is lots of equipment, noise and alarms, and there may also be distressed relatives and

**Table 2.5  Critical care/intensive therapy unit: specific considerations**

| | |
|---|---|
| General | • Monitor ABC carefully throughout the assessment and focus on patient stability |
| Database | • History of accident (if appropriate) and investigations with results following admission<br>• Note all injuries, any surgery that may have been required and any equipment that may limit how you perform your assessment, e.g. external fixators<br>• Are spinal precautions being taken? If so all patients will be treated as unstable until proven otherwise, and this should be clearly documented. If you are not sure, treat as unstable |
| CNS | • If there is any suspicion of head trauma it is very important to monitor conscious levels |
| CVS | • Be vigilant for any signs of deterioration, loss of stability or impending circulatory shock |
| Renal | • Fluid balance is important to identify patients at risk of shock |
| RS | • Consider the mode of any ventilation and method of delivery, e.g. ETT or tracheostomy and note ventilator settings<br>• RR: include set rate (from ventilator) and spontaneous rate (if the patient is doing some breathing on their own) |
| MS | • Note any limitations secondary to other injuries, e.g. positioning if spinal precautions being taken<br>• Be aware of any potential loss of ROM– may need to consider splinting<br>• Be aware of skin condition as this can have an impact on what you are able to do. The nursing staff are an invaluable source of information! |

ABC, airway, breathing, circulation; ETT, endotracheal tube; ROM, range of movement; RR, respiratory rate.

distressing situations. However, it is the environment where there is the most support because the patients are closely monitored and there is a high ratio of nurses to patients.

- Do not be too distracted by the technology in the bed area and do not forget that there is a patient in the bed! However, appreciate that you will have to be reliant on technology to gain information for your assessment as many patients will not be able to communicate effectively.
- As part of your assessment, it is important to identify appropriate physiotherapy problems, but also to recognize that, for some patients, treatment will not be indicated. Just because a patient

is on a ventilator (life support machine) it does not necessarily mean that enthusiastic respiratory physiotherapy is required!
- Be prepared for the possibility that you may have to make very quick decisions when a patient is deteriorating or becoming critically unstable. This may mean that you cannot carry out the assessment as originally intended because you may need to respond immediately to the changing circumstances.

> **Top tip!**
> If any alarms go off when you are at the bedside on ITU, alert nursing or medical staff immediately. NEVER touch any buttons!

## 2.6 MEDICAL PATIENTS (Table 2.6)

- Most admissions are due to exacerbations of long-standing conditions, such as chronic obstructive pulmonary disease. Your main focus is to identify physiotherapy problems such as breathlessness, sputum retention and respiratory failure.

| Table 2.6 | Medical patient: specific considerations |
|---|---|
| Database | • Establish a baseline of the patient's 'usual' values as these may not be within the 'normal' range because of the patient's underlying long-term condition<br>• Determine the extent of any deterioration since previous admission/assessment and discuss the likely prognosis as this may affect your choice of active physiotherapy treatment and/or the use of NIV |
| CVS | • Be alert for any symptoms (e.g. bilateral ankle swelling) of right heart failure (cor pulmonale), which is a common complication of COPD |
| RS | • For patients in respiratory failure you may also include an assessment for NIV<br>• Psychological factors are very important, e.g. the extent to which anxiety may be affecting breathlessness (see 3.8 Breathlessness (dyspnoea) scales)<br>• Once the initial acute illness is addressed, you need to explore the factors that may have led to this acute episode. Investigate self-management strategies, such as inhaler technique, chest clearance at home, managing breathlessness, compliance with medication and smoking cessation |

COPD, chronic obstructive pulmonary disease; NIV, non-invasive ventilation.

## 2.7 GOAL-ORIENTED ASSESSMENT (Table 2.7)

- Ask patients what their main problems/issues are and what they would like to achieve from therapy.
- Discuss and agree a manageable number of patient-centred goals and work with patients to put these into a list of priorities.
- For each goal identify:
  - how much the patient can already do towards it
  - how difficult it is to attempt it now
  - how the patient feels about their ability now
  - a documented target date for achievement of the goal (interim goals may also need to be identified)

### Table 2.7 Factors to be considered in goal-oriented assessment

| | |
|---|---|
| Musculoskeletal/ neurological | • Pain<br>• Reduced range of movement<br>• Muscle weakness<br>• Loss of balance or coordination<br>• Sensory loss/altered sensation<br>• Loss of function<br>• Reduced exercise tolerance |
| Respiratory | • Increased work of breathing, breathlessness<br>• Reduced lung volumes<br>• Sputum retention |
| Psychological/ cognitive | • Anxiety<br>• Depression<br>• Motivation<br>• Self-efficacy<br>• Knowledge about condition and its management<br>• Confusion |
| Social | • Home environment<br>• Family and friends<br>• Education<br>• Work (employment)<br>• Basic economic transactions<br>• Economic self-sufficiency<br>• Recreation and leisure<br>• Community life |
| Other factors | • Other medical problems |

- factors that may need to be addressed to enable patients to achieve their goal
- factors that may be addressed by physiotherapy and those requiring a referral to other members of the health and social care team.
- For physiotherapy-related problems, such as functional, musculoskeletal and respiratory problems, carry out further assessment as appropriate. Assess the patient's suitability for pulmonary rehabilitation and refer if appropriate.
- For further detail regarding goal-oriented assessment, see Further reading.

## 2.8 FUNCTIONAL ASSESSMENT

### RANGE OF MOVEMENT

- Check for any problem with range of movement (ROM) (ask patients, as well as observing their movement during functional activity).
- Using a table (such as Table 2.8) within your notes can be useful (insert 'Full' or 'Reduced' as appropriate).
- If limited, complete a musculoskeletal ROM assessment at affected joints.

**Table 2.8  Range of movement**

|  | Range of movement |  |
|---|---|---|
| Head |  |  |
| Trunk and pelvis |  |  |
| **Upper limb** | Right | Left |
| Shoulder region |  |  |
| Elbow |  |  |
| Wrist and hand |  |  |
| **Lower limb** | Right | Left |
| Hip |  |  |
| Knee |  |  |
| Foot and ankle |  |  |

## MUSCLE STRENGTH

- Check for any muscle weakness or signs of wasting.
- Again, a table such as Table 2.9 may be used (insert 'Full' or 'Reduced' as appropriate).
- If there is any weakness that limits function, assess muscle strength of affected muscles (see 3.41 muscle charting (Oxford grading)).

**Table 2.9 Muscle strength**

| Muscle strength | Right | Left |
|---|---|---|
| Upper limb | | |
| Lower limb | | |

## SENSATION

- Check for any history of sensory or proprioceptive loss. If necessary, follow with a detailed check of sensation and/or proprioception (see 3.21 Dermatomes).

## BALANCE/COORDINATION

- Check for any history of falls or any obvious lack of coordination when moving. If necessary, complete a detailed balance assessment.

## FUNCTIONAL MOBILITY

- Assess the following functions (stopping at the stage that is appropriate, e.g. if the patient cannot move from sitting to standing, do not proceed to standing or walking) – see Table 2.10.

**Table 2.10 Functional mobility assessment**

| | Usual ability | Current ability |
|---|---|---|
| Movement<br>Bed mobility (move up bed) | | |
| Rolling (to side lying) | | |
| Side lying to sitting | | |
| Sitting to standing | | |

|  | Usual ability | Current ability |
|---|---|---|
| Standing balance | | |
| Walking on level ground | | |
| Walking up a hill | | |
| Walking on uneven ground | | |
| Exercise tolerance (*state distance walked*) | | |
| Stairs | | |
| Wheelchair mobility (if appropriate) | | |
| Self-propel chair | | |
| Transfer | | |
| **Self-care and domestic activities** Washing | | |
| Personal grooming | | |
| Toileting | | |
| Dressing | | |
| Eating | | |
| Drinking | | |
| Looking after own health (e.g. taking medication and knowing what it is for) | | |
| Safety awareness in home | | |
| Shopping | | |
| Preparing meals | | |
| Housework and laundry | | |

- Many hospitals use forms/tables to document progress; Table 2.10 is an example. Insert 'Independent', 'Requires supervision', 'Requires help' or 'Not possible'.

## 2.9 ACUTE COMMUNITY PATIENT ASSESSMENT

Table 2.11 lists appropriate considerations for patients in the community. The reader is also referred back to Fig. 1.5 (see page 7).

### Table 2.11 Acute community patient assessment

| | |
|---|---|
| **Check medical stability** <br> Is patient sufficiently medically stable to remain in community environment? | • Is required medical support available, e.g. oxygen therapy, regular observations? <br> • What is risk of medical deterioration/relapse? Any risk factors, e.g. age, significant co-morbidities? <br> • Can/will patient rapidly receive help if they deteriorate, e.g. rapid response teams, regular district nurse visits? <br> • Do they need further complex medical intervention or treatment, e.g. scans/CXR/ABGs? Does this require admission to hospital? <br> • Is medication optimized? Can prescribed medication be delivered at home? (e.g. intravenous antibiotics may require admission to hospital, depending on locality) |
| **Check functional ability** <br> Does the patient have sufficient functional stability to remain in the community environment? | • Is patient's mobility safe/can it be made safe to allow them to be alone for periods? (e.g. moving the bed downstairs if patient is unable to manage stairs) <br> • Would equipment help? e.g. commode <br> • How will the patient get food and drink? <br> • How will they get help if they need it? Do they have access to a phone and/or pull cord alarm? <br> • How will the patient wash/dress? |
| **Social circumstances** <br> Does the patient have sufficient social support to remain in the community environment? | • Who does the patient live with? Do they live alone? <br> • What type of accommodation does the patient live in? <br> • Does the patient need to use stairs, e.g. for bed/toileting? <br> • Do they have any social support in place already, e.g. social services, meals, local family/neighbours? <br> • Does the patient own the property? <br> • What local services are available? Where can you find out? Are they 24 hours/office hours only? |

- Is the patient able to manage their medications/operate delivery devices effectively? Are any medications new/unfamiliar? Would this compromise safety at home?
- What acute support is available in the community and what hours are they available?
  - Intermediate care teams
  - Hospital at home teams
  - Admission avoidance schemes
  - Community matrons
  - Specialist multidisciplinary teams

ABG, arterial blood gas; CXR, chest x-ray.

## FURTHER READING

Bovend'Eerdt, T.J., Botell, R.E., Wade, D.T., 2009. Writing SMART rehabilitation goals and achieving goal attainment scaling: a practical guide. Clin. Rehabil. 23, 352.

# CHAPTER 3

# Assessment tools

- 3.1 Arterial Blood Gases (ABGs)  25
- 3.2 Attachments  34
- 3.3 Auscultation  36
- 3.4 AVPU  42
- 3.5 Blood Pressure (BP)  44
- 3.6 Blood Results  49
- 3.7 Breathing Pattern (See under 3.54 Respiratory Pattern – Page 148)
- 3.8 Breathlessness (Dyspnoea) Scales  56
- 3.9 Capillary Refill Test  58
- 3.10 (Invasive) Cardiac Monitoring  59
- 3.11 Central Venous Pressure (CVP)  62
- 3.12 Cerebral Perfusion Pressure (CPP)  64
- 3.13 Chest Drains  65
- 3.14 Chest Imaging (Including Chest X-rays)  68
- 3.15 Chest X-ray (See under 3.14 Chest Imaging – Page 68)
- 3.16 Chest Wall Shape  74
- 3.17 (Digital) Clubbing  77
- 3.18 Consent  78
- 3.19 Cough Assessment  79
- 3.20 Cyanosis  81
- 3.21 Dermatomes  82
- 3.22 Drugs  84
- 3.23 Early Warning Scores (EWS)  90
- 3.24 Electrocardiogram (ECG) (See under 3.35 Heart Rhythms – Page 109)
- 3.25 Electrolytes (See under 3.6 Blood Results – page 49)
- 3.26 End-Tidal Carbon Dioxide ($ETCO_2$)  92
- 3.27 Exercise (aerobic fitness) Testing  95
- 3.28 Exercise Tolerance  101
- 3.29 $FEV_1$/FVC (See under 3.40 Lung Volumes and Lung Function Tests – Page 120)
- 3.30 Flow Volume Loops (See under 3.40 Lung Volumes and Lung Function Tests – Page 120)
- 3.31 Fluid Balance (Including Urine Output)  102
- 3.32 General Observation (See Chapter 1)
- 3.33 Glasgow Coma Scale (GCS)  105
- 3.34 Heart Rate (HR)  107
- 3.35 Heart Rhythms  109

# ASSESSMENT TOOLS

3.36 Inspiratory Muscle Testing (See under 3.40 Lung Volumes and Lung Function Tests – Page 120)
3.37 Intracranial Pressure (ICP)   116
3.38 ITU (critical care) Charts   119
3.39 Level of Consciousness   120
3.40 Lung Volumes and Lung Function Tests (Pulmonary Function Tests)   120
3.41 Muscle Charting (Oxford Grading)   125
3.42 Myotomes   127
3.43 Oxygen Delivery   129
3.44 Pain Score   134
3.45 Palpation   135
3.46 Peak Flow (See under 3.40 Lung Volumes and Lung Function Tests – Page 120)
3.47 Percussion Note   137
3.48 Pulse Oximetry   139
3.49 Pupils   141
3.50 Quality of Life Questionnaires   142
3.51 Rating of Perceived Exertion (RPE)   144
3.52 Reflexes   146
3.53 Renal Function (See under 3.6 Blood Results and 3.31 Fluid Balance – Pages 49 and 102)
3.54 Respiratory Pattern   148
3.55 Respiratory Rate (RR)   151
3.56 Resuscitation Status   152
3.57 Sedation/Agitation Score   154
3.58 Sputum Assessment   156
3.59 Surgical Incisions   157
3.60 Swallow Assessment   159
3.61 TPR (Temperature, Pulse and Respiration) Chart   160
3.62 Ventilation–Perfusion (V/Q) Matching   164
3.63 Ventilator Observations   166
3.64 Work of Breathing   169

This chapter contains assessment procedures that may be used with respiratory patients. For each assessment performed, you need to select those that are most appropriate for each patient. If you are unsure which are appropriate, refer back to the assessment checklists in Chapter 2, which relate the tools to the assessment process.

There are many texts available that briefly discuss assessment tools. This book aims to cover these techniques in a standardized format. It gives a simple, step-by-step explanation of exactly how they are performed and how to interpret the findings.

Each technique has distinct sections:

- *Definition*: explains what the tool or measurement is about in simple terms.

- *Purpose*: suggests why the test/measurement is done and why this is important for physiotherapists.
- *Procedure*: gives step-by-step instructions on how the technique should be undertaken.

> NB: In all instances it is assumed that hands are washed, the procedure has been explained to the patient and that suitable consent has been obtained (and documented).

- *Findings*: looks at the findings and how this information may be of use to you, linking theoretical concepts to practical application.
- *Documentation*: demonstrates how this information should be recorded in your notes.

> NB: In all instances it is assumed that the entry is dated and timed.

Literature and clinical practice vary widely; therefore, each assessment tool is based on a consensus of identified articles, key texts and clinical experience. In line with other titles in this series, an amalgamation of evidence style has been taken to allow for a standardization of the text. Specific texts and examples of further reading are at the end of each assessment tool as appropriate. For ease of use, this chapter is in alphabetical order. Please note that many of these procedures are referred to using different terminology depending on your work setting and location.

## 3.1 ARTERIAL BLOOD GASES (ABGs)

### DEFINITION
Analysis of an arterial blood sample to measure the levels of oxygen (partial pressure of oxygen ($P_aO_2$) and oxygen saturations ($S_aO_2$)), carbon dioxide (partial pressure of carbon dioxide ($P_aCO_2$)), pH, bicarbonate ($HCO_3^-$) levels and base excess (BE). Blood gases can also be taken from a venous or capillary sample.

### PURPOSE
An arterial blood gas (ABG) is used to determine the significance of any respiratory or metabolic compromise, monitor deterioration and identify respiratory failure. This can provide information to guide treatment with oxygen therapy and/or ventilatory support. It may be used as an outcome measure following physiotherapy treatment and to aid clinical reasoning and treatment selection.

## PROCEDURE

Physiotherapists need to be able to analyse the results (Fig. 3.1.1). The procedure itself involves taking an arterial blood sample and is normally carried out only by medical or nursing staff and some extended scope physiotherapists with specialized training.

### RADIOMETER ABL 700 SERIES

ABL725
PATIENT REPORT      Syringe – S 195µL      Sample #

**Identifications**
Patient ID
Patient Last Name
Patient First Name
Sample Type              Arterial
temp.                         37.0°C

**Blood Gas Values**

| | | | | | |
|---|---|---|---|---|---|
| pH | 7.461 | | [ | - | ] |
| $pO_2$ | 18.0 | kPa | [ | - | ] |
| $pCO_2$ | 5.04 | kPa | | | |

**Oximetry Values**

| | | | | | |
|---|---|---|---|---|---|
| ctHb | 11.5 | g/dL | [ | - | ] |
| $sO_2$ | 98.8 | % | [ | - | ] |
| $FO_2Hb$ | 95.0 | % | [ | - | ] |
| FCOHb | 1.0 | % | [ | - 1.5 | ] |
| FHHb | 1.2 | % | [ | - | ] |
| ↑FMetHb | 2.8 | % | [ | - 1.5 | ] |

**Electrolyte Values**

| | | | | | |
|---|---|---|---|---|---|
| $cK^+$ | 3.6 | mmol/L | [ | 3.4 - 5.0 | ] |
| $cNa^+$ | 14.2 | mmol/L | [ | 135 - 145 | ] |
| $cCa^{2+}$ | 1.12 | mmol/L | [ | - | ] |
| $cCa^{2+}(7.4)_c$ | 1.16 | mmol/L | [ | - | ] |
| $cCl^-$ | 107 | mmol/L | [ | 98 - 107 | ] |

**Metabolite Values**

| | | | | | |
|---|---|---|---|---|---|
| cGlu | 6.8 | mmol/L | [ | 3.0 - 8.0 | ] |
| cLac | 0.6 | mmol/L | [ | 0.5 - 1.6 | ] |

**Temperature Corrected Values**

| | | |
|---|---|---|
| pH(T) | 7.461 | |
| $pCO_2(T)$ | 5.04 | kPa |
| $pO_2(T)$ | 18.0 | kPa |

**Oxygen Status**

| | | |
|---|---|---|
| $ctO_{2c}$ | 15.6 | Vol% |
| $p50_e$ | 3.24 | kPa |

**Acid Base Status**

| | | |
|---|---|---|
| $cBase(Ecf)_c$ | 3.0 | mmol/L |
| $cHCO_3^-(Pst)_c$ | 27.2 | mmol/L |

**Notes**
↑   Value(s) above reference range
c   Calculated value(s)
e   Estimated value(s)

**Fig 3.1.1** Example of a set of arterial blood gas results. As can be seen, a blood gas result may contain more information than blood gases alone.

## 3.1 Arterial blood gases (ABGs)

### FINDINGS (Fig. 3.1.2, Table 3.1.1)

You should also consider haemoglobin (Hb) levels when interpreting ABG results (see 3.48 Pulse oximetry). Fig 3.1.2 summarizes the process of interpreting ABG's in flowchart format.

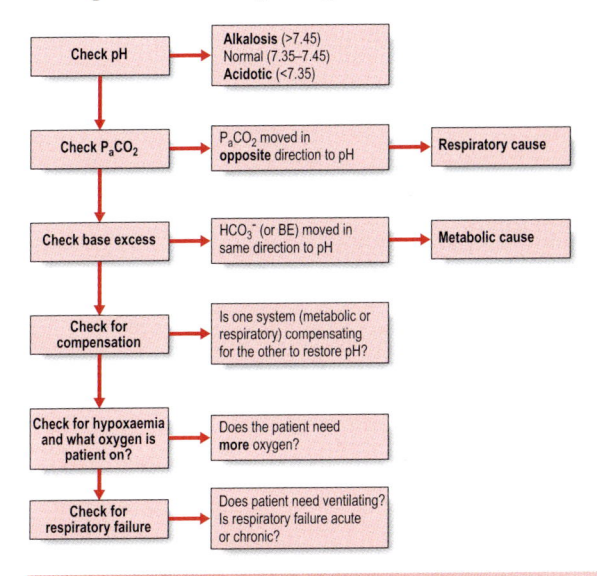

```
Check pH  →  Alkalosis (>7.45)
             Normal (7.35–7.45)
             Acidotic (<7.35)

Check P_aCO_2  →  P_aCO_2 moved in           →  Respiratory cause
                  opposite direction to pH

Check base excess  →  HCO_3^- (or BE) moved in  →  Metabolic cause
                      same direction to pH

Check for compensation  →  Is one system (metabolic or
                           respiratory) compensating
                           for the other to restore pH?

Check for hypoxaemia  →  Does the patient need
and what oxygen is       more oxygen?
patient on?

Check for            →  Does patient need ventilating?
respiratory failure     Is respiratory failure acute
                        or chronic?
```

**Fig 3.1.2** Flowchart for arterial blood gas analysis.

**Table 3.1.1 Blood gas measurements**

| | |
|---|---|
| pH | Measure of level of acidity or alkalinity of blood<br>Normal range 7.35–7.45 |
| $P_aCO_2$ | Partial pressure of carbon dioxide in arterial blood (plasma)<br>Normal range 4.7–6 kPa (35–45 mmHg) |
| $P_aO_2$ | Partial pressure of oxygen in arterial blood (plasma)<br>Normal range 10.7–13.3 kPa (80–100 mmHg) |
| $S_aO_2$ | Saturation level of Hb in arterial blood (measures how fully saturated each unit of Hb is, given as a percentage)<br>Normal range 95–100% |
| $HCO_3^-$ | Amount of bicarbonate (base) in the blood<br>Normal range 22–26 mmol l$^{-1}$ |
| BE (base excess) | Base excess is a simpler way of expressing bicarbonate levels and gives the amount of $HCO_3^-$ above or below the average value of 24 mmol l$^{-1}$<br>Normal range −2 to +2 |

NB. Partial pressure refers to the pressure exerted by one specific gas (e.g. oxygen), which forms part of the total pressure exerted by the mixture of gases (e.g. oxygen, carbon dioxide and nitrogen) in the blood.

**Process of Interpreting ABGs.**
1. **Check pH**
   a. Decide whether pH is within normal range or whether there is an acidosis (low pH below 7.35) or an alkalosis (high pH above 7.45).
   b. Anything outside the normal range can interfere with metabolism and may become critical. Discuss any recent changes with medical or nursing staff.
2. **Check $P_aCO_2$**
   If there is an acidosis or an alkalosis, you need to decide whether this is due to a respiratory or metabolic problem. Identify any hypercapnia (high $P_aCO_2$ above 6 kPa) or hypocapnia (low $P_aCO_2$ below 4.7 kPa) (Box 3.1.1).
   i. Respiratory acidosis is when hypercapnia causes the blood to become more acidic (i.e. high $P_aCO_2$ and low pH).
   ii. Respiratory alkalosis is when hypocapnia causes the blood to become more alkalotic (i.e. low $P_aCO_2$ and high pH).

---

**Box 3.1.1**

**Example of respiratory acidosis**
- pH          7.20
- $P_aCO_2$   8.3 kPa
- $P_aO_2$    8.4 kPa

**Example of respiratory alkalosis**
- pH          7.49
- $P_aCO_2$   4.2 kPa
- $P_aO_2$    15.0 kPa

---

➔ *Top tip!*
If there is a respiratory problem the pH and $P_aCO_2$ tend to see-saw (e.g. if the pH is higher than normal, the $P_aCO_2$ would be lower than normal).

---

Hypercapnia suggests that the patient is hypoventilating (underbreathing). This may be due to fatigue or neuromuscular weakness, so the patient may need support with ventilation, e.g. non-invasive ventilation (NIV). Hypercapnia may also be due to insensitivity to high $P_aCO_2$ levels, as seen in some patients with chronic obstructive pulmonary disease (COPD) ($CO_2$ retainers).

Hypocapnia suggests that the patient is hyperventilating (overbreathing). This may be due to pain or anxiety. The patient may need reassurance and might benefit from a pain review, or breathing control and relaxation techniques (see 3.55 Respiratory rate).

3. **Check $HCO_3^-$ (or BE)**

    Identify whether the patient has a high or low bicarbonate (or BE). Higher values (above 26 mmol l$^{-1}$ or BE >+2) will make the blood more alkaline, whereas lower values (below 22 mmol l$^{-1}$ or BE <−2) will make the blood more acidic. Either of these can, therefore, be used to determine the metabolic (i.e. non-respiratory) contribution to the pH (Box 3.1.2).

---

**Box 3.1.2**

**Example of metabolic acidosis**
- pH           7.28
- $HCO_3^-$    14 mmol l$^{-1}$
- BE           −8

**Example of metabolic alkalosis**
- pH           7.5
- $HCO_3^-$    30 mmol l$^{-1}$
- BE           +8

---

**➡ Top tip!**
If there is a metabolic problem the pH and the $HCO_3^-$ move in the same direction as if in an elevator (e.g. if the pH is high the $HCO_3^-$ will also be high).

---

i. Metabolic acidosis is when lower levels of bicarbonate (or BE) cause the pH to become more acidic (both change in the same direction to become lower).

ii. Metabolic alkalosis is when higher levels of bicarbonate (or BE) cause the pH to become more alkaline (both change in the same direction to become higher).

## 4. Check for compensation

Compensation is the balancing of one system with the other (respiratory and metabolic) to make sure the pH stays within normal limits. This is very important for metabolism. Each system (respiratory or metabolic) can therefore adjust its levels of carbon dioxide or bicarbonates in response to changes in the other system. For example, if there is a respiratory acidosis, the kidneys can start to conserve bicarbonates in the blood (i.e. not pass as many out in the urine). This will raise $HCO_3^-$ levels and make the blood more alkaline, thereby restoring the pH.

> **Top tip!**
>
> If the pH and the $P_aCO_2$ have moved in the same direction, this suggests that the respiratory system is compensating and the problem is metabolic.
>
> If the pH and the $HCO_3^-$ have moved in the opposite direction, this suggests that the metabolic system is compensating and the problem is respiratory.

The respiratory system can react to change quickly (within a couple of hours) but the metabolic system may take approximately 2 days to respond. Any compensation may be full (complete) or partial (Box 3.1.3).

---

**Box 3.1.3**

**Example of a fully compensated respiratory acidosis**
- pH          7.36
- $P_aCO_2$   8.4
- $HCO_3^-$   28
- BE          +4

**Example of a partially compensated metabolic acidosis**
- pH          7.32
- $P_aCO_2$   4.2
- $HCO_3^-$   16
- BE          −6

---

i. Full compensation is seen when both the $P_aCO_2$ and the $HCO_3^-$ are outside the normal range and the pH is within the normal range.
ii. Partial compensation is when the $P_aCO_2$ and $HCO_3^-$ are both out of range but the pH is not quite within normal limits.

Note that it may be impossible to distinguish between compensated respiratory acidosis and compensated metabolic alkalosis, or between compensated respiratory alkalosis and compensated metabolic acidosis without looking at other clinical findings or a series of ABGs.

The chart in Table 3.1.2 assumes that any compensation is complete not partial.

**Table 3.1.2 Respiratory and metabolic acidosis and alkalosis**

| Status | pH | $P_aCO_2$ | $HCO_3^-$ |
|---|---|---|---|
| Normal | 7.35–7.45 | 4.7–6 | 22–24 |
| Respiratory acidosis | ↓ | ↑ | Normal |
| Metabolic acidosis | ↓ | Normal | ↓ |
| Compensated respiratory 'acidosis' | Normal | ↑ | ↑ |
| Compensated metabolic 'acidosis' | Normal | ↓ | ↓ |
| Respiratory alkalosis | ↑ | ↓ | Normal |
| Metabolic alkalosis | ↑ | Normal | ↑ |
| Compensated respiratory 'alkalosis' | Normal | ↓ | ↓ |
| Compensated metabolic 'alkalosis' | Normal | ↑ | ↑ |

5. **Check oxygenation**

   **Hypoxaemia.** $P_aO_2$ reflects the ability of the lungs to allow the transfer of oxygen from the environment to the circulating blood. A reduced $P_aO_2$, regardless of $F_iO_2$ (how much oxygen the patient is receiving), is called hypoxaemia. You should always check if a reading has been taken while the patient is receiving oxygen therapy, and, if so, how much they are receiving (see 3.43 Oxygen delivery). A $P_aO_2$ of 10.7 kPa is normal, but would not be considered normal if the patient is receiving 60% oxygen.

   Identify any significant, deteriorating or potentially critical levels of hypoxaemia. In acute respiratory disease, a $P_aO_2$ <10.7 kPa may be significant and <7.3 kPa may be critical, but chronic respiratory patients may be able to tolerate lower oxygen levels, and hypoxaemia may not be considered significant until it drops below 7.3 kPa. Oxygen therapy should be considered for patients with significant (or worsening) hypoxaemia.

   $S_aO_2$ levels may be used to determine the need for oxygen therapy. Give oxygen when $S_aO_2$ <90% (see 3.48 Pulse oximetry).

6. **Check for respiratory failure**
   a. Identify whether the patient is in respiratory failure – is it type I or type II?

i. Type I respiratory failure occurs when $P_aO_2$ is low and $P_aCO_2$ is normal or slightly reduced.
ii. Type II respiratory failure occurs when $P_aO_2$ is low and $P_aCO_2$ is high.

b. Acute or chronic respiratory failure?

Identify whether any respiratory failure is acute, chronic or a mixture of the two. Respiratory failure of recent onset, or deteriorating, should be discussed with a senior as oxygen therapy or ventilation may be urgently required.

> *Top tip!*
> Type One failure is when One gas (i.e. Oxygen) is affected – remember they both begin with O!
>
> Type Two is when Two gases (i.e. oxygen and carbon dioxide) are affected.

When respiratory failure is due to acute respiratory disease, there may be little or no compensation from raised $HCO_3^-$ levels because it takes time (e.g. days) for adequate compensation to occur. Therefore, the pH is likely to be low (respiratory acidosis).

When respiratory failure is due to a chronic respiratory disease there may be compensation from raised $HCO_3^-$ levels. Therefore, the pH may be normal, or only slightly lower than normal (compensated respiratory acidosis). Check any current ABG results against any previous or usual results as this will also help to confirm the diagnosis of acute or chronic failure.

It is important to identify the extent to which any respiratory failure is acute or chronic because patients with chronic respiratory disease can tolerate lower levels of hypoxaemia and may not need oxygen therapy until their levels become lower. Additionally, they may be reliant on a 'hypoxic' drive to breathe, and if they are given too much oxygen therapy their drive to breathe could be seriously reduced.

## DOCUMENTATION

Record each value together with time and date of test, and any oxygen therapy or ventilation support given at the time of measurement. Record the patient's position if appropriate.

## CLINICAL EXAMPLES (ANSWERS FOLLOW)

### Case 1
A 65 year old man enters the Accident and Emergency Department short of breath. He has no chest pain but a productive cough. His ABGs are reflected below. What do these show? Can you suggest a possible cause?

- pH             7.29
- $P_aO_2$       8.2
- $P_aCO_2$      8.4
- $HCO_3^-$      24
- BE             1

### Case 2
A 16 year old girl is about to go to theatre for removal of her tonsils. She has no previous medical history (PMH) but is extremely anxious. Her ABGs immediately before her operation are shown below. What do they show and what is the possible explanation?

- pH             7.49
- $P_aO_2$       10
- $P_aCO_2$      3.9
- $HCO_3^-$      22
- BE             −2

### Case 3
An 80 year old ex-miner presents with these ABGs. What do they show? Would you be concerned about these results? What is the reason for your decision?

- pH             7.39
- $P_aO_2$       9.9
- $P_aCO_2$      7.2
- $HCO_3^-$      32
- BE             6

### Case 4
A 25 year old man with no PMH was admitted with a history of frequent urination, excessive thirst and nausea for the past 3 days. He was drowsy but coherent and his breathing was notably deep. What do his ABGs show? Would you take any action to try to affect his breathing?

- pH             7.1
- $P_aO_2$       17
- $P_aCO_2$      2.5
- $HCO_3^-$      3.5
- BE             −24

## ANSWERS TO CLINICAL EXAMPLES
### Case 1
This man has a respiratory acidosis (uncompensated). It is an acute condition and may be due to pneumonia or a severe chest infection – note he has type II respiratory failure and may require additional ventilator support.

### Case 2
This girl has respiratory alkalosis (uncompensated). This is an acute situation and has been caused by hyperventilation due to anxiety.

### Case 3
This man has compensated respiratory acidosis. This is a chronic situation because there has been enough time for $HCO_3^-$ to increase and his pH is within the normal range, despite his high $P_aCO_2$ (remember he is an ex-miner; therefore, respiratory disease would not be uncommon).

### Case 4
This man has partially compensated metabolic acidosis. His symptoms suggest diabetes, which can cause a fall in $HCO_3^-$ and therefore a fall in pH. There is some compensation because the $P_aCO_2$ has gone down, suggesting that he is breathing more in order to try and raise the pH. This is only partially successful because his pH is still below the normal range. Physiotherapy is not going to help his breathing at this point as he needs medical attention to stabilize his diabetes.

## 3.2 ATTACHMENTS

### DEFINITION
These may be any piece of equipment that is attached to the patient, e.g. intravenous (i.v.) lines, central venous line, ECG lines, surgical drains, ventilator tubing, saturations monitor and catheter (Figs 3.2.1 and 3.2.2).

### PURPOSE
The purpose of an attachment is specific to what is being monitored – many of these will be discussed throughout this chapter. However, the ultimate aim of attachments can be subdivided as:

- monitoring/assessment of the patient, e.g. saturations monitor, intracranial pressure (ICP) bolt
- provision or drainage of fluids, i.e. what is going in and out, such as drips and drains
- treatment/support of the patient, e.g. renal support, ventilator.

## 3.2 Attachments

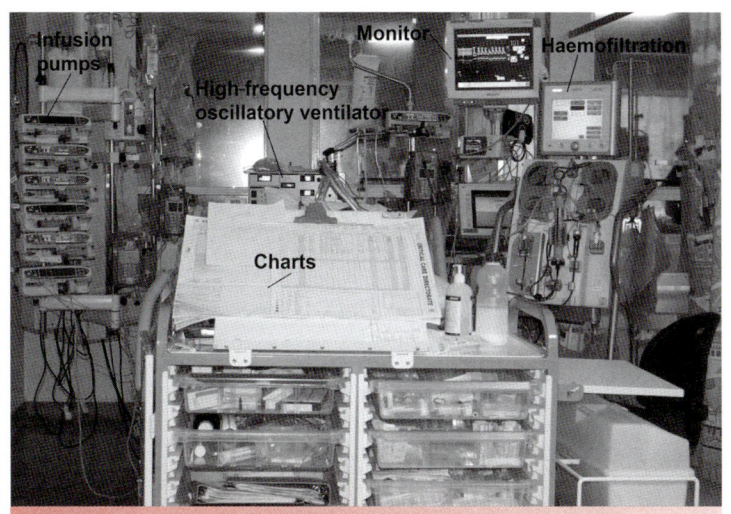

**Fig 3.2.1** Example of patient attachments in an intensive therapy unit.

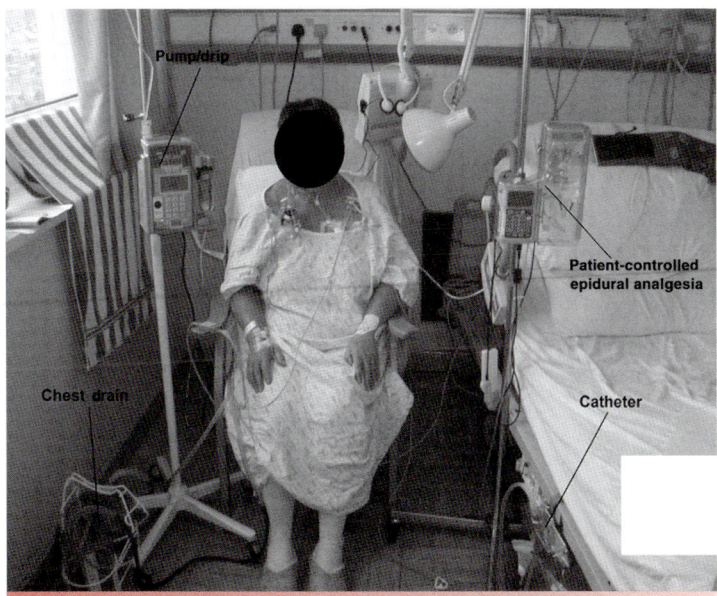

**Fig 3.2.2** Example of patient attachments in the ward setting.

## ASSESSMENT TOOLS

### PROCEDURE
Be aware of all attachments and take care not to displace any equipment during your assessment.

### FINDINGS
If you do not know what a piece of equipment or fluid running into the patient is, ask the nursing staff. It may be important information that will influence what you can/cannot do with the patient, e.g. changing position.

### DOCUMENTATION
As part of your assessment, all attachments should be noted within your documentation.

## 3.3 AUSCULTATION

### DEFINITION
Auscultation is the process of using a stethoscope to listen to and interpret the lung/breath sounds generated by airflow through the airways.

### PURPOSE
This assessment technique can help identify sputum retention in the airways, or areas of atelectasis. It may be used as an outcome measure before and after physiotherapy. It can also help identify deterioration or more serious pathology such as a pneumothorax that may need further medical investigation.

### PROCEDURE
- Equipment
  - Good quality stethoscope (Fig. 3.3.1).
  - Sterilizing wipes.

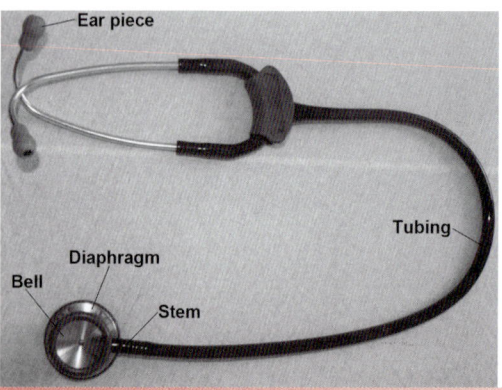

**Fig 3.3.1** Labelled diagram of a stethoscope.

## 3.3 Auscultation

- Method
  - Clean the diaphragm and earpieces with wipes.
  - Place earpieces in your ears (earpieces should face forwards in order to fit into your auditory canals).
  - Check that the stethoscope is tuned to the diaphragm (tap the diaphragm lightly – can you hear this clearly? If not twist the metal connector until you can hear the tapping sound most clearly).
  - Ask the patient if they would be willing to remove any items of clothing in order to expose the chest area, providing this is appropriate and you can maintain their dignity and comfort.
  - Position the patient so you can access anterior and posterior aspects of the chest, e.g. sitting up over the edge of the bed or sitting forwards in a chair. If they are confined to bed, you may need help to sit them forwards slightly when listening posteriorly or help them to roll into side lying. Note that you may have to access the posterior segments by moving your stethoscope under the patient if they are very unwell and unable to move.
  - Warn the patient to inform you if they start to feel dizzy.
  - Place the stethoscope firmly on the chest wall in the positions described in Fig. 3.3.2 and Table 3.3.1.
  - Listen during both inspiration and expiration. Listen to each zone of the lungs on alternate sides of the chest to compare your findings.

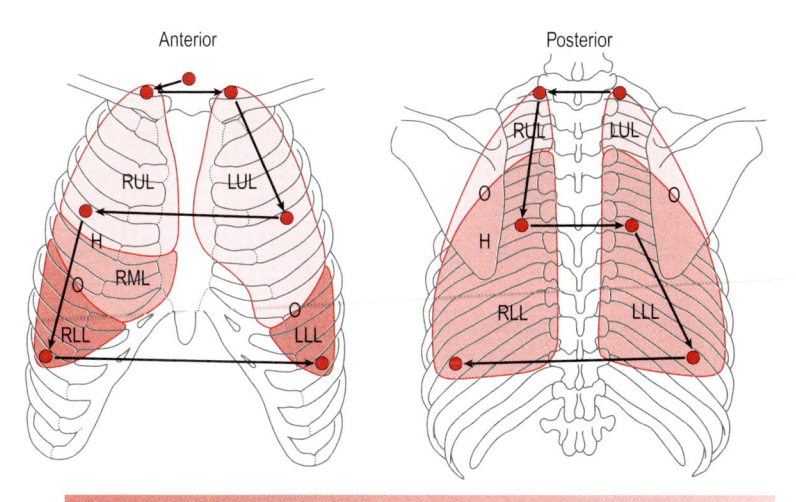

**Fig 3.3.2** Auscultation points.
Reproduced and modified with kind permission from Pryor JA, Prasad SA. 2008 Physiotherapy for Respiratory and Cardiac Problems, 4th Edn. Edinburgh, UK: Churchill Livingstone.

H, horizontal fissure; LLL, left lower lobe; LUL, left upper lobe; RLL, right lower lobe; RUL, right upper lobe; RML, right middle lobe.

## ASSESSMENT TOOLS

**Table 3.3.1  Auscultation zones**

| Anterior | Apical | Left and right |
| --- | --- | --- |
|  | Middle | Left and right |
|  | Lower | Left and right |
| Mid-axillary |  | Left and right |
| Posterior | Upper | Left and right |
|  | Middle | Left and right |
|  | Lower | Left and right |

- Make sure you listen to one or two full breaths in AND out at each point.
- Allow the patient a period of rest or normal breathing between zones or if they become dizzy.
- When you have finished, note your findings and clean your stethoscope.

### FINDINGS

For each zone, record whether breath sounds are normal or bronchial, loud or quiet, and then identify any added sounds.

Breath sounds (Table 3.3.2) arise in the trachea and bronchi and are caused by the turbulence of the air as it flows in and out of

**Table 3.3.2  Breath sounds**

| **Normal breath sounds**<br>Soft, muffled, louder on inspiration, fade in expiration, ratio 1:2 | Turbulence in the large airways |
| --- | --- |
| **Bronchial breathing**<br>Expiration louder and longer with pause between inspiration and expiration (sounds like Darth Vader)<br>Heard normally over trachea | If heard over lung fields, suggests:<br>• Consolidation<br>• Collapse without a plug<br>• May also be heard at the lip of a pleural effusion |
| **Breath sounds quiet or absent?**<br>Poor air entry<br>Low lung volumes<br>Atelectasis | May be due to:<br>• Shallow breathing<br>• Poor positioning<br>• Collapse with complete obstruction of airway<br>• Sounds filtered by air (hyperinflation)<br>• Sounds filtered by pleura, chest wall (obese or muscular patients, pleural effusion, pneumothorax, haemothorax)<br>• Pneumothorax |

## 3.3 Auscultation

these large airways. If you listen over the trachea (just below the cricoid cartilage or Adam's apple) you will hear what they sound like at the source. You will notice that they are very loud here and also quite harsh sounding. Inspiration and expiration are heard clearly (both are loud) and there is a very slight pause between them. These sounds are known as bronchial breath sounds because they are generated in the bronchi (and trachea).

- **Normal breath sounds.** If you listen anywhere over the lung fields (including all of the zones shown in Fig. 3.3.2) the sounds are much quieter because you are over lung parenchyma and the air in the lungs has absorbed a lot of the sound. This attenuates the sound, making it smoother, gentler and more continuous, so it is harder to tell when inspiration changes to expiration. Since we expect to hear these sounds when auscultating over the lungs we call them 'normal breath sounds'.
- **Bronchial breathing** (bronchial breath sounds heard over lung fields). If you are listening over the lungs and what you hear sounds loud, harsh and discontinuous (i.e. like bronchial breath sounds), it is not 'normal' and suggests that these sounds have not been dampened down by the air in the lungs – usually because in that area of lung the air has been replaced by something solid (consolidated). A solid area transmits sound very well because it vibrates more than air (ask the patient to say '99' while auscultating and the sound will be very clear over consolidated lung tissue). These sounds may occur over an area of lobar pneumonia where the alveoli fill with clotted inflammatory exudate, or over collapsed lung tissue (occurring without a sputum plug), or at the lip of a pleural effusion.
- **Breath sounds quieter than normal.** If the breath sounds are very quiet it might be because the patient is very large and therefore the sounds have been dampened down by excess soft tissue. Make sure you press the stethoscope firmly to the chest wall and press through the adipose tissue to get the best sound transmission. It might, however, be because the breaths were quite small and not generating much turbulence. Perhaps the patient is not breathing very deeply? Does this fit with your observation and palpation? Is one side of the chest moving more than the other side?

> *Top tip!*
> Think! If a patient is not breathing very deeply – what possible implications might this have and what problems might this cause?

- **Absent breath sounds.** A pleural effusion, sputum plugging or pneumothorax could prevent sounds from being heard by absorbing the sound completely before it can be transmitted to the chest wall.

> **Top tip!**
> If you auscultate and hear a 'silent' chest, it may mean that the patient is in extremis and is unable to move air at all (check airway and stethoscope). This is a medical emergency and you need to seek expert medical assistance straight away!

- **Breath sounds louder than normal.** Loud breath sounds suggest more turbulence in the large airways. This is usually due to obstruction or narrowing of these airways, e.g. due to COPD. Narrower airways are harder to breathe through, so the patient may be working harder in order to breathe.
- Other added sounds.
  – **Crackles** (Table 3.3.3)

**Table 3.3.3 Added sounds: crackles**

| Crackles | Short, non-musical, popping sounds, fine or coarse | |
|---|---|---|
| **Fine crackles** Reopening of airways sounds like rubbing hair next to your ear | Atelectasis | • Short, explosive<br>• Periphery lung<br>• Reduce with deep breath |
| | Intra-alveolar oedema | • 'Tissue paper'<br>• Do not resolve with deep breath or cough<br>• Late inspiration (NB: interstitial fibrosis) |
| | Secretions small airways | • High pitched<br>• Peripheral<br>• Clear with cough |
| **Coarse crackles** Sounds like pouring milk on rice crispies | Obstruction more proximal and larger airways with sputum. May be inspiratory as well as expiratory | • Early expiratory: central airways<br>• Late expiratory: more peripheral airways<br>• Large deep sound<br>• Changes/clears with coughing |

## 3.3 Auscultation

- **Fine crackles.** Sound like rubbing a hair next to your ear. They may be due to pulmonary oedema or sputum but are often caused by the sudden opening of small airways when lung volumes are low, suggesting atelectasis. If it is the latter, they often resolve after some deep breathing exercises.
- **Coarse crackles.** Sound like rice crispies crackling as you add the milk. They may be caused by sputum, particularly if you notice that they reduce or change after coughing.

> **Top tip!**
> Remember crackles are only heard if the velocity of airflow is adequate and breath sounds are audible. Coarse crackles move/disappear when the patient coughs, whereas fine crackles remain the same after coughing.

- **Wheezes** (Table 3.3.4). Whistling sounds due to narrowed airway walls vibrating against each other, indicating airway obstruction. High-pitched wheeze indicates bronchospasm or oedema in the walls of conducting airways. Low-pitched wheeze indicates sputum.

You should identify whether wheezes or crackles are heard during inspiration or expiration and whether they are heard early or late during the breath. Louder sounds heard early in the breath are more likely to be generated centrally (in the larger airways).

- **Pleural rub** (Table 3.3.5). A sound like boots crunching on snow suggests that the pleura are inflamed.

| Table 3.3.4 | Added sounds: wheezes | |
|---|---|---|
| Wheezes | Musical sounds due to vibration of wall of narrowed airway | |
| *High pitched* | Bronchospasm | • Potential increased work of breathing |
| *Low pitched* | Sputum | • Disrupted turbulent flow<br>• Change with coughing |
| *Localized* | Tumour<br>Foreign body | • Limited to a local area on auscultation |

## Table 3.3.5 Other sounds

|  | Sounds like | Cause |
|---|---|---|
| **Pleural rub** | • Creaking/rubbing (like boots on snow)<br>• Localized/generalized<br>• Soft/loud<br>• Equal inspiration to expiration | • Inflammation of pleura<br>• Infection<br>• Tumour |
| **Stridor** | • Constant pitch on inspiration and expiration<br>• Produced in upper airways | • Croup<br>• Laryngeal tumour<br>• Upper airway obstruction<br>! Alert medical staff as the patient's airway is at great risk of compromise |

– **Stridor** (Table 3.3.5). This is a sound like a loud 'barking' noise. Occurs during both inspiration and expiration and is usually caused by significant upper airway obstruction, which could be a foreign body or tumour. If stridor is heard as a new/recent symptom, alert the medical staff immediately as the patient's airway could be compromised.

> *Top tip!*
> Auscultation is only a small part of respiratory assessment and its interpretation is subjective. Always consider your findings alongside other assessment information before drawing any firm conclusions.

### DOCUMENTATION

Record the patient's position and your findings, e.g. 'Normal breath sounds heard in all zones, quieter in right base. Coarse crackles in right base on mid-expiration, reduced after coughing'.

## 3.4 AVPU (SEE ALSO 3.33 GLASGOW COMA SCALE AND 3.39 LEVEL OF CONSCIOUSNESS)

### DEFINITION

AVPU is a simple test to give an indication of the level of arousal of a patient. It is a quick neurological assessment and the acronym stands for Awake, Voice, Pain and Unresponsive.

## 3.4 AVPU

### PURPOSE

This was adapted from paediatric practice to acute adult care as a method of quickly identifying change in neurological arousal. While effective, it does not replace formal neurological assessment such as the Glasgow Coma Scale (see 3.33 Glasgow Coma Scale and 3.57 Sedation/agitation score).

### PROCEDURE

There are only four possible outcomes within this scale. Ask the patient a simple question such as 'hello – can you hear me'. Look for the best response in the patient. If the patient is asleep, he or she should be woken first. It is not valid in patients who are sedated or having paralyzing drugs.

1. *Alert.* The patient is alert and responsive and answers clearly and coherently. The patient could be sitting up reading the paper or talking to visitors.
2. *Voice.* The patient is responding only to voice commands and may be drowsy, possibly keeping eyes closed and not speaking coherently. There is a response to your voice. Does the patient wake up when you call their name? This response may be only a grunt.
3. *Pain.* The patient responds only to pain. To elicit any response from the patient requires a painful stimulus (for procedure and appropriate painful stimuli, see 3.33 Glasgow Coma Scale).
4. *Unresponsive.* The patient is unresponsive. This patient is unresponsive or unconscious. They may be in a 'coma' with no eye opening or movement.

### FINDINGS

Note that you are looking for a change in status. If a patient who was previously alert is now only responding to voice, this is a significant change and should be notified to the team. Any patients who are only responding to pain or who are unresponsive warrant an urgent medical review.

### DOCUMENTATION

This should be documented in the neurological section of the assessment as the level of response according to the first letter of the acronym, e.g. 'The patient was at "V" on the AVPU scale'. Some units write down the acronym AVPU and circle the appropriate letter e.g. AVP☺

## 3.5 BLOOD PRESSURE (BP)

***DEFINITION***

The force exerted by the blood against the walls of the arteries. Blood pressure (BP) can be measured in a large artery (e.g. brachial or femoral), and may be measured invasively through an arterial line or non-invasively through a cuff and sphygmomanometer (manually) or by using an automated BP machine (Figs 3.5.1 and 3.5.2).

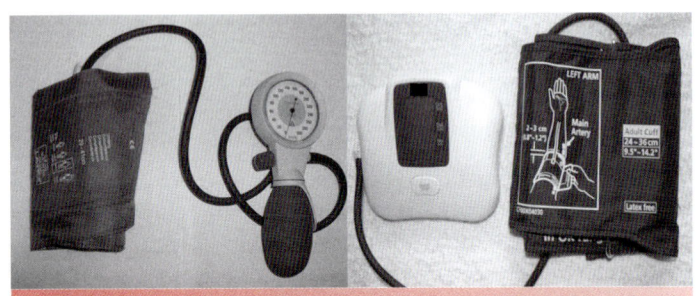

**Fig 3.5.1** Non-invasive blood pressure monitors. Manual sphygmomanometer (left) and automated blood pressure machine (right).

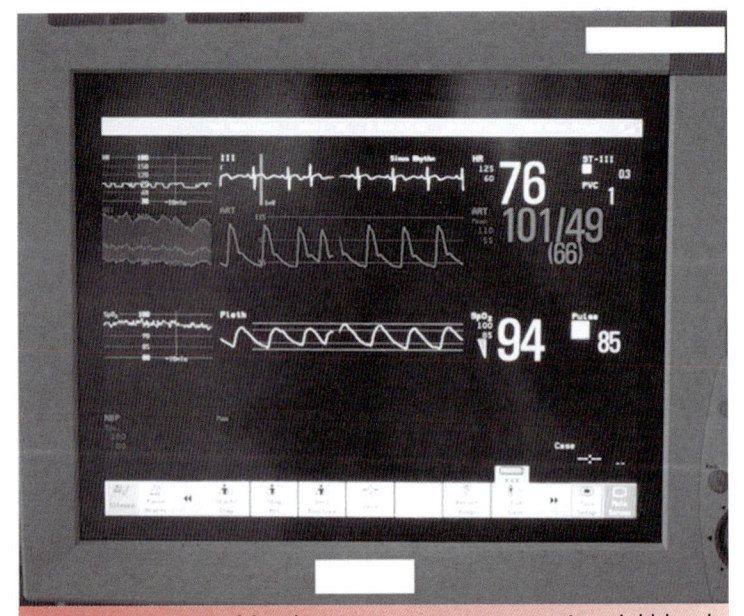

**Fig 3.5.2** Invasive blood pressure measurement. Arterial blood pressure trace; the arterial trace is second from the top with a blood pressure of 101/49 and a mean arterial pressure of 66.

### 3.5 Blood pressure (BP)

#### PURPOSE

The measurement of BP is very important when determining cardiovascular status and stability in the critically ill patient as well as monitoring patients at risk of deterioration that could lead to circulatory failure. The physiotherapist must also take BP status into account when standing and mobilizing patients and when prescribing exercise. BP may also be used as an outcome measure for physiotherapy treatment.

#### PROCEDURE

##### Non-invasive BP monitoring: cuff and sphygmomanometer (Fig. 3.5.3)

- Choose an appropriate sized cuff for the patient (Table 3.5.1). The inflatable part of the cuff should go round at least 75% of the arm circumference, but it should not be any longer than the arm circumference.
- Observe the patient's arm carefully throughout the procedure. If there is any pain or numbness or if the arm starts to change colour, becoming blue or purple, the cuff should be immediately deflated and removed from the arm.
  1. The patient should be sitting still with their elbow extended and supported at approximately the level of the heart. Ideally, the patient should rest for 5 minutes before the measurement is taken.

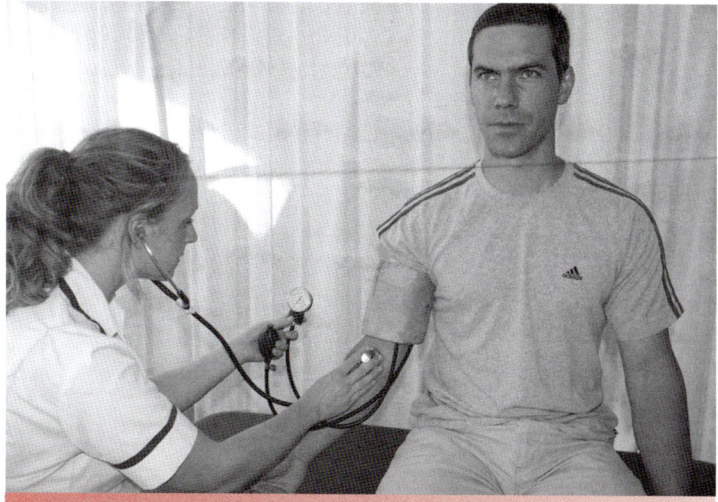

**Fig 3.5.3** Blood pressure measurement using a sphygmomanometer.

## ASSESSMENT TOOLS

Table 3.5.1  Blood pressure cuff sizes

| Size of cuff | Upper arm circumference (measure at mid-point of humerus) |
| --- | --- |
| Child/small adult cuff | <23 cm |
| Standard/regular adult cuff | <33 cm |
| Large adult cuff | <50 cm |
| Adult thigh cuff | <53 cm |

2. Explain that the cuff will exert an uncomfortable pressure for a few seconds while inflated.
3. Ensure there is no residual air in the cuff (squeeze any air out), then wrap the cuff around the arm above the elbow joint so that the 'arterial point' on the cuff is over the brachial artery (medial to the biceps muscle on the anterior aspect).
4. Fasten the cuff firmly but not too tightly.
5. Inflate the cuff to a pressure higher than the 'likely' systolic pressure. For most people 150 mmHg will be sufficient; however, if a person is known to have a high BP, or if you are measuring following exercise, you will need to inflate to a higher pressure, up to a maximum of 260 mmHg.
6. Release the pressure in the cuff slowly while using a stethoscope over the brachial artery pulse at the anterior aspect of the elbow. Listen for the sounds generated by the blood flow in the artery. These are described as soft knocking or pounding sounds (Korotkoff sounds).
7. Record the pressure when you FIRST hear the knocking sounds. This is the systolic pressure.
8. Record the pressure when you STOP hearing the knocking sounds. This is the diastolic pressure.
9. Release the valve and allow the cuff to completely deflate before removing it from the patient's arm.
10. Check the arm to ensure circulation (normal pink colour) is restored and no damage has been caused.

### Cuff and automated BP machine *(Fig. 3.5.4)*

- Make sure you are familiar with the machine and any manufacturer's instructions before commencing.

## 3.5 Blood pressure (BP)

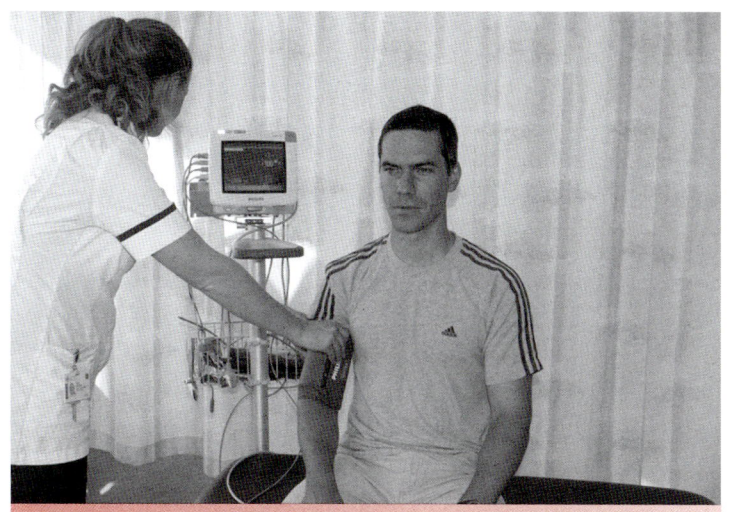

**Fig 3.5.4** Measuring blood pressure using an automated machine.

- Carry out steps 1–5 above; then press the start button on the automated BP machine.
- It is very important to observe the patient's arm carefully. If there is any pain or numbness or if the arm starts to change colour, becoming blue or purple, the cuff should be immediately deflated and removed from the arm.
- If the machine stays inflated too long, or continually reinflates over and over again, stop the procedure and check the patient's circulation.
- Check the arm to ensure circulation (normal pink colour) is restored and no damage has been caused.

### FINDINGS

Average resting BP is 120/80 mmHg. The first figure (120 mmHg) represents the systolic pressure, achieved during ventricular contraction. The second figure (80 mmHg) is the diastolic pressure, achieved during ventricular diastole. Invasive measurements of BP will also calculate MAP (mean arterial pressure) (see 3.10 (Invasive) Cardiac monitoring).

Normal BP ranges between 95/60 and 140/90 mmHg, but does tend to increase with age. The significance of any 'abnormal' values (i.e. outside the range given) depends on what is usual for that patient. A one-off abnormal measurement may not be significant, because BP varies with many factors, including activity levels, emotion (including stress!) and temperature. It is more important to look at the 'trend' and identify any changes over time. However, if there is a sudden significant change in BP you should seek senior advice.

Hypotension is defined as BP <95/60 mmHg (adults). If BP is dropping over time, or is below the patient's usual level, this could be significant because it could compromise blood flow to the brain, leading to fainting or, in more serious situations, circulatory failure and death. A patient whose pulse is higher than their systolic BP at rest is likely to be significantly compromised and may require urgent attention and circulatory support (e.g. intravenous fluids and possibly cardiopulmonary resuscitation (CPR)).

Postural hypotension may occur if the BP drops when the patient sits or stands up, leading to dizziness or fainting. Patients are most at risk when getting out of bed for the first time after a period of bed rest. If the patient's BP is low, take extra care when getting them up and ensure that this is carried out slowly.

Hypertension is defined as BP >140/90 mmHg. The significance of high BP depends on the patient's age and their usual values. A diastolic pressure of >95 mmHg warrants a degree of caution with any 'active' treatments or mobilization. Any unexplained increase in BP above the normal range and the patient's usual values should be referred to the medical practitioner for investigation.

> ***Top tip!***
> If the BP is much higher than the heart rate or much lower than the heart rate seek advice from a senior as this can indicate an acute problem.

Blood pressure should also be considered in conjunction with any medication the patient may be on that may affect the BP:

- Inotropes (e.g. adrenaline, noradrenaline, enoximone, milrinone) help to increase BP. Patients who need this support are less stable, and need extra caution with physiotherapy techniques.

- Anti-hypertensives (e.g. beta-blockers, angiotensin-converting enzyme inhibitors, diuretics) help to reduce BP and may affect the patient's response to exercise (see 3.22 Drugs).

## DOCUMENTATION
Record measurement, e.g. resting BP on L arm in sitting using (name of) machine = 120/80 mmHg.

## 3.6 BLOOD RESULTS

### DEFINITION
There are a number of different types of blood tests; Table 3.6.1 summarizes those that are particularly relevant to physiotherapists. Other types of blood tests include those for immunology and virology.

### PURPOSE
Blood results reflect body systems and how they are functioning. They may give an indication of deterioration or improvement. Some results can be markers of specific problems. For example, they can be used to identify patients:

- developing a chest infection which might require chest physiotherapy
- at risk of bleeding and the need for caution with manual chest therapy techniques
- at risk of deep vein thrombosis (DVT) and caution with mobilization
- with anaemia who may be at risk of low oxygen levels.

Table 3.6.1 Types of blood tests relevant to physiotherapists

| Haematology | Biochemistry | Blood sciences | Microbiology |
|---|---|---|---|
| Full blood count Coagulation | CRP Lactate Liver function U&Es Cardiac markers (ABGs) | Glucose | Identification of bacterial infections |

ABG, arterial blood gas; CRP, C-reactive protein; U&Es, urea and electrolytes.

## ASSESSMENT TOOLS

### PROCEDURE

Blood tests in the main are carried out by medical and nursing staff. Some specialist physiotherapists may take some blood samples, e.g. ABGs.

### FINDINGS

> **Top tip!**
> There is much variation in the normal values referenced by different texts, online and in hospitals. Therefore, the ranges provided here are guides; when reviewing patient results the normal values used in your own facility should be used.

### Full blood count

A common test that assesses the state of health of the patient (Table 3.6.2). For definitions, see the further reading suggested at the end of this section.

### Coagulation screen *(Table 3.6.3)*

This gives an indication of the body's ability to form clots. Activated prothrombin time (APTT) and prothrombin time (PT) are often tested together to evaluate the function of all clotting factors. PT is often adjusted to the international normalized ratio (INR), especially in the assessment of anticoagulant therapy (blood thinners). Fibrinogen assesses the body's ability to form and break down clots.

### C-reactive protein (CRP)

CRP (Table 3.6.4) is an inflammatory marker (often used alongside the white blood count). It serves as a general marker of infection and inflammation.

### Lactate

Lactate (Table 3.6.4) is a by-product of anaerobic respiration and rises in patients with sepsis. It is also a marker of the severity of stress response. Hyperlactataemia is a mild-to-moderate persistent increase in blood lactate concentration (2–5 mmol $l^{-1}$) without metabolic acidosis. Lactic acidosis is a persistently increased blood lactate level (usually >4–5 mmol $l^{-1}$) in association with metabolic acidosis. It is not within the remit of this book to discuss lactic acidosis; see Further reading on this subject at the end of this section.

## 3.6 Blood results

**Table 3.6.2 Full blood count results**

| Test (normal range) | Too high | Too low |
|---|---|---|
| (WBC) (4–11 × 10⁹/l) | May be increased with infections, inflammation, cancer, leukaemia | Decreased with some medications (e.g. chemotherapy), when immune system is compromised, some severe infections, bone marrow failure |
| WBC differentials, i.e. neutrophils, lymphocytes, monocytes, eosinophils and basophils | Measures the percentage of each type of WBC in blood. A low level is generally due to immunocompromise. Neutropenia is a low neutrophil count and happens after chemotherapy; neutropenic sepsis is when the patient becomes very unwell and has no reserves to fight off infection ||
| RBC (M = 4.5–6.5 × 10¹²/l) (F = 3.9–5.6 × 10¹²/l) | Increased when too many made and with fluid loss, e.g. diarrhoea, dehydration or burns | Decreased with anaemia; may mean patients tire easily as reduced RBC and Hb reduce oxygen-carrying ability |
| Hb (M = 13.5–18.0 g/dl) (F = 11.5–16.0 g/dl) | Mirrors RBC results ||
| Hct (M = 42–54%) (F = 38–46%) | Mirrors RBC results ||
| MCV (76–96 fl) | Increased with $B_{12}$ and folate deficiency | Decreased with iron deficiency and disorders of Hb |
| Platelets (150–400 × 10⁹/l) | May be increased in people living at altitude. Myeloproliferative disorder may cause greater propensity for DVT and clotting problems. Oestrogen and the oral contraceptive pill can cause increased levels | Decreased when greater numbers used, e.g. bleeding, some inherited disorders, leukaemia and chemotherapy. Caution with treatment as high risk of bleeding |

DVT, deep vein thrombosis; F, female; Hb, haemoglobin; Hct, haematocrit; M, male; MCV, mean corpuscular volume; RBC, red blood cell; WBC, white blood cell.

### Table 3.6.3 Coagulation results

| Test (normal range) | Too high | Too low |
|---|---|---|
| APTT (25–35 s) PT (11–15 s) INR (0.8–1.2) | Clotting deranged, bleeding time prolonged and interventions may have higher risk of bleeding; many treatments can be contraindicated. Check with senior! | Potential hypercoagulable state in which blood may clot too easily; this is unusual but could lead to, for example, DVT |
| Fibrinogen (2.0–4.0 g/l) | May rise sharply in any condition that causes inflammation or tissue damage. Rise will increase a person's risk of developing a blood clot | Low levels impair the body's ability to form a stable clot; may be an inherited disorder or can be the result of illness. Caution with treatment and discuss with senior! |
| Platelets | See Full blood count | |

APTT, activated prothrombin time; DVT, deep vein thrombosis; INR, international normalized ratio; PT, prothrombin time.

### Table 3.6.4 C-reactive protein and lactate results

| Test | Too high | Very high |
|---|---|---|
| CRP Normally <6 mg/l | Acute infection or inflammation | A CRP >100 mg $l^{-1}$ is suggestive of bacterial infection |
| Lactate Normally 0.5–1.8 mmol/l | Gives an indication of anaerobic respiration | Levels of 4–5 in presence of metabolic acidosis = lactic acidosis, i.e. your patient is very unwell! |

CRP, C-reactive protein.

## 3.6 Blood results

**Table 3.6.5 Urea and creatinine results**

| Test | Measurement significance |
|---|---|
| Urea (2.1–8.0 mmol/l) | Urea is the final degradation product of proteins and amino acid metabolism and is the most important catabolic pathway for eliminating excess nitrogen in the body. Blood loss, fluid balance, renal failure and liver failure can also cause rises in urea |
| Creatinine (M = 80–115 µmol/l) (F = 70–100 µmol/l) | A waste product produced by muscles; related to muscle mass (women and children tend to have lower levels). Creatinine blood levels can also increase temporarily as a result of muscle injury and are generally slightly lower during pregnancy. Creatinine clearance measures how well creatinine is removed from your blood by your kidneys. It is completed using a blood sample and 24 hour urine collection |

F, female; M, male.

### Urea and electrolytes (U&Es)

U&Es (Table 3.6.5) encompass renal function and electrolyte tests. Urea and creatinine are the main markers of renal function.

Electrolytes are salts that conduct electricity and are found in the body fluid, tissue and blood (e.g. chloride, calcium, magnesium, phosphate, sodium and potassium). Sodium ($Na^+$) is concentrated in the extracellular fluid (ECF) and potassium ($K^+$) is concentrated in the intracellular fluid. Proper balance is essential for muscle coordination, heart function, fluid absorption and excretion, nerve function and concentration. Levels may be affected by diet, total body water and the amount of electrolytes excreted by the kidney.

### Sodium ($Na^+$)

$Na^+$ (Table 3.6.6) plays a vital role in maintaining the concentration and volume of the ECF. It is the main cation of the ECF and a major determinant of ECF osmolality. $Na^+$ is important in maintaining irritability and conduction of nerve and muscle tissue and assists with the regulation of acid–base balance.

**Table 3.6.6** Sodium and potassium results

| Test | Too high | Too low |
|---|---|---|
| Sodium (135–145 mmol/l) | Hypernatraemia >145 mmol l$^{-1}$ Caused by disruption in water balance: either too little going in or too much coming out, or by salt loading | Hyponatraemia <135 mmol l$^{-1}$ caused by water intoxication, altered ADH secretion and drugs, e.g. diuretics and MDMA (ecstasy). If seen in dehydrated patients, seek expert help |
| Potassium (3.5–5.0 mmol/l) | Hyperkalaemia >5.5 mmol l$^{-1}$ (severe is >7 mmol l$^{-1}$) Decreased or impaired potassium excretion most common in renal failure but also potassium-sparing diuretics and specific inherited diseases | Hypokalaemia <3.5 mmol l$^{-1}$ Caused by renal losses, GI losses and drug effects (commonly diuretics) |
| | If potassium is out of range in either direction there is a high risk of cardiovascular instability, especially if the patient suffers from renal failure! If you are unsure if it is appropriate to treat, seek senior advice! ||

ADH, antidiuretic hormone; GI, gastrointestinal.

### *Potassium (K⁺)*

K$^+$ (Table 3.6.6) is the major ion of the body. Nearly 98% of potassium is intracellular, with the concentration gradient maintained by the sodium- and potassium-activated adenosine triphosphatase pump. The ratio of intracellular to extracellular potassium is important in determining the cellular membrane potential.

Small changes in the extracellular potassium level can have profound effects on the function of the cardiovascular and neuromuscular systems.

Other electrolytes have different functions but are not as commonly reviewed by physiotherapists and therefore will not be covered here.

## Cardiac markers

These are substances released into the bloodstream when the heart is damaged. The two commonly used markers are troponin and creatinine kinase. These can be used to diagnose, evaluate and monitor heart problems.

## Glucose

Blood sugar levels are important in maintaining acid–base balance in the body. It has previously been suggested that tight glycaemic control improved mortality, but this is currently under question. However, glucose levels (Table 3.6.7) are important because altered results may cause dramatic effects and yet can be easily treated.

| Table 3.6.7 Glucose results | | |
|---|---|---|
| **Test** | **Too high** | **Too low** |
| Glucose Normal 3.6–6 mmol/l | Hyperglycaemia leads to fatigue and thirst. In the diabetic patient when high levels have been present for some time, diabetic ketoacidosis can develop – a medical emergency | Hypoglycaemia Sympathetic responses: sweating, tremors and tachycardia CNS symptoms of confusion convulsions, dizziness and syncope |

CNS, central nervous system.

## Microbiology

The pathology department can run specific tests for infections within the blood. If bacteria are identified, an appropriate antibiotic can be prescribed. Specific tests will not be discussed within this text.

## DOCUMENTATION

Blood results relevant to your assessment should be documented within the cardiovascular system (CVS) section of your assessment or under a heading of haematology. It is good practice to identify the trends of the results and note any cautions to treatment based upon these.

## FURTHER READING

Skinner, S., 2005. Understanding Clinical Investigations: A Quick Reference Manual, 2nd edn. Balliere Tindall, London, UK.

## 3.7 BREATHING PATTERN
## (See under 3.54 RESPIRATORY PATTERN – page 148)

## 3.8 BREATHLESSNESS (DYSPNOEA) SCALES

### DEFINITION
Breathlessness (dyspnoea) is the subjective sensation of difficulty in breathing or the perception of an increased effort to breathe. There are several different tools that may be used to 'measure' this perception by attempting to quantify what is essentially a qualitative patient experience. Two scales that are commonly used by physiotherapists are:

- Borg breathlessness scale (CR10)
- Medical Research Council (MRC) scale.

Other breathlessness scales include visual analogue scales, the baseline dyspnoea index (BDI) and scales found within other quality of life measurement questionnaires such as the St Georges questionnaire and chronic respiratory questionnaire.

### PURPOSE
Breathlessness scales have a number of uses:

- The Borg scale (CR10) can be used to rate exercise intensity during an exercise test and identify an appropriate level of intensity when prescribing exercise or activity. It may also be used to monitor progress during an exercise programme and as a guide when patients are learning to desensitize themselves to their breathlessness.
- The MRC scale can be used to classify patients according to the functional impact of their respiratory disease. This can be used to monitor progression or deterioration and in helping to select patients who are appropriate for pulmonary rehabilitation and medical interventions.
- Breathlessness scales can also be used as outcome measures for drug therapy and for physiotherapy interventions such as exercise programmes, breathing control or sputum clearance.

### PROCEDURE
#### Borg scale *(Table 3.8.1)*
Ensure that the patient understands the scale points and descriptors; then ask them to rate how strong their feeling of breathlessness is at that moment according to the criteria.

## 3.8 Breathlessness (dyspnoea) scales

**Table 3.8.1  The Borg CR10 scale**

| Number | Strength of perception of breathlessness |
|---|---|
| 0 | Nothing at all |
| 0.3 | Extremely weak (just noticeable) |
| 0.5 | |
| 0.7 | Very weak |
| 1 | Weak |
| 2 | |
| 2.5 | Moderate |
| 3 | |
| 4 | |
| 5 | Strong (heavy) |
| 6 | |
| 7 | Very strong |
| 8 | |
| 9 | |
| 10 | Extremely strong (almost maximal) |
| * | Absolute maximum/highest possible |

Note that some texts refer to the absolute maximum level of breathlessness as above 10; on some adapted scales, this may be marked with a symbol, e.g. '*'. There is also a Borg scale that uses 20 points (see 3.51 Rating of perceived exertion).

### MRC scale *(Table 3.8.2)*

Ask the patient to pick the statement that is most applicable to them. If their breathlessness is variable, they should focus on the past 2 weeks when answering.

### FINDINGS
### Borg scale

As this is a subjective measure, patient ratings will vary considerably and we cannot compare patients with each other using this scale. Patients are generally encouraged to try and exercise at between 3 and 5 on the scale and to learn to pace themselves accordingly. Patients who get more breathless than '5' during exercise or activity should be monitored carefully, but, providing their sensation

## ASSESSMENT TOOLS

**Table 3.8.2  Medical Research Council (MRC) scale**

| MRC score | Descriptor |
| --- | --- |
| 1 | I only get breathless with strenuous exercise |
| 2 | I get short of breath when hurrying on the level or walking up a slight hill |
| 3 | I walk slower than other people of the same age on the level because of breathlessness, or I have to stop for breath when walking at my own pace on the level |
| 4 | I stop for breath after walking about 100 yards or after a few minutes on the level |
| 5 | I am too breathless to leave the house or garden by myself (i.e. I can only leave the house if I am with others and/or need a car to get out) |

of effort is back to resting levels within 5 minutes of stopping, they are generally considered safe to exercise at that intensity.

### MRC scale

Some pulmonary rehabilitation programmes use MRC grade 3 and above as a criterion for inclusion in a pulmonary rehabilitation programme, as this indicates that the patient is limited by their breathlessness and may find benefit from such a programme.

### DOCUMENTATION

For the Borg scale, record the score and state whether at rest or during exercise. Record the intensity of any exercise undertaken and any additional (qualitative) comments the patient may make about their breathlessness.

For the MRC scale, record the score and note the status of the patient (i.e. whether or not the patient has had a recent exacerbation or whether he or she is in a stable condition).

### FURTHER READING

Borg, G. The Borg CR10 Scale®. © G. Borg, 1982, 1998, 2004. Borg Perception, Gunnar Borg, Rädisvägen 124, S-165 73 Hässelby, Sweden.

Stenton, C., 2008. The MRC breathlessness scale. Occup. Med. 58, 226–7.

## 3.9 CAPILLARY REFILL TEST

### DEFINITION

A quick test performed on the nail beds to monitor dehydration and the amount of blood flow to tissue.

## PURPOSE

This test is used to assess the amount of blood flow to the tissue and to determine the patient's tissue perfusion. If capillary refill is slower than expected then reduced cardiac output or impaired digital perfusion is suspected and should be further investigated by medical staff.

## PROCEDURE

- This should be performed at the level of the heart.
- Pressure is applied to the nail bed until it turns white, indicating that the blood has been forced from the tissue (blanching).
- Once the tissue has blanched, pressure is removed.
- The time taken for the tissue to return to its normal colour is then recorded.
- The tissue should normally take less than 2 seconds to return to its normal colour.

## FINDINGS

A slow capillary refill time may indicate dehydration (hypovolaemia), hypothermia, peripheral vascular disease or sepsis. If the slow refill time is caused by dehydration the patient may potentially have dry tenacious secretions, which are difficult to expectorate.

A fast capillary refill time may indicate overhydration (hypervolaemia). This may have an impact on physiotherapy if the patient shows other signs of symptoms of fluid overload leading to pulmonary oedema. Capillary refill time can also be very fast if the patient is very hot and is vasodilated to lose heat.

## DOCUMENTATION

Capillary refill time should be recorded (especially if greater than 2 seconds) under the cardiovascular section of your assessment.

## 3.10 (INVASIVE) CARDIAC MONITORING

### DEFINITION

Invasive cardiac monitoring comprises the calculation of cardiac activity and cardiac function through the insertion of invasive (intravascular) catheters.

### Key terminology

- *Stroke volume index*: a calculation relating the stroke volume (the amount of blood pumped by the left ventricle in one contraction) to the body surface area (normal range = 33–47 ml/$m^2$/beat).

- *Cardiac index*: a calculation that relates the cardiac output (stroke volume × heart rate) to body surface area (normal range = 2.5–4.0 l/min/m$^2$).
- *Global ejection fraction*: the proportion of the volume of blood in the ventricles at the end of diastole that is ejected during systole; it is the stroke volume divided by the end-diastolic volume, often expressed as a percentage (normally range = 65 ± 8%).
- *Mean arterial pressure*: the average BP in an individual. It is not a true average as diastole counts twice as much as systole because two-thirds of the cardiac cycle is spent in diastole (normal range = 70–105 mmHg). It is calculated using the equation:

$$MAP = [(2 \times diastolic) + systolic] / 3$$

- *Systemic vascular resistance*: the resistance to flow that must be overcome to push blood through the circulatory system (normal range = 800–1200 dynes.sec/cm$^5$).

## PURPOSE

The purpose of invasive cardiac monitoring is to quickly ascertain how the heart is functioning, and to help assess the cardiovascular status of a patient. Information gained from these devices provides information on cardiac function and assists in the optimization of cardiac function as well as in the treatment of heart failure, kidney failure, pulmonary disease and complex fluid management. Such devices will be seen within the intensive therapy unit (ITU) and theatre environments.

For physiotherapists, cardiac monitoring will assist in the assessment of the cardiovascular system. This will aid in deciding whether physiotherapy treatment is required and whether the patient is likely to tolerate any intervention. If a patient has any form of invasive cardiac monitoring it should be observed throughout the treatment, and, if gross changes occur, treatment should be stopped immediately (e.g. sudden reductions in BP). In these circumstances, medical advice must be sought.

## PROCEDURE

The insertion of all invasive cardiac monitoring is completed by specifically trained doctors.

### Arterial pressure

Intra-arterial pressure measurement is performed through the insertion of a line into an artery (this is called an arterial line). Arterial BP is then interpreted through a transducer and displayed on the monitor system.

## 3.10 (Invasive) Cardiac monitoring

### *Central venous pressure (CVP)*

Reflects right ventricular filling and is usually monitored via a catheter which sits within the superior vena cava. The catheter is usually inserted via the subclavian vein within the thorax or the internal jugular vein. Less commonly, central venous catheters can be inserted via the femoral vein (see 3.11 Central venous pressure).

### *Pulmonary artery catheter (Swan–Ganz)*

A pulmonary artery catheter is a catheter which is inserted into a pulmonary artery. This is done by a video-fluoroscopy-guided catheter that is passed via a major vein (e.g. internal jugular vein) through and into the right atrium and right ventricle. From here, the catheter can be forwarded into one of the pulmonary arteries. It is a diagnostic tool used to detect heart failure or sepsis.

Pulmonary artery occlusion pressure (previously known as wedge pressure) can also be recorded using a pulmonary artery catheter by passing a balloon-tipped catheter into a pulmonary capillary. The normal range for pulmonary artery occlusion pressure is 2–12 mmHg.

### *Continuous thermodilution (e.g. PiCCO®)*

The PiCCO® system (Pulsion Medical Systems AG; Fig. 3.10.1) requires the insertion of a thermodilution catheter in the femoral or axillary artery and a central venous catheter (no catheter in right atrium required). By using a complex technique of transpulmonary thermodilution the monitor is able to provide specific

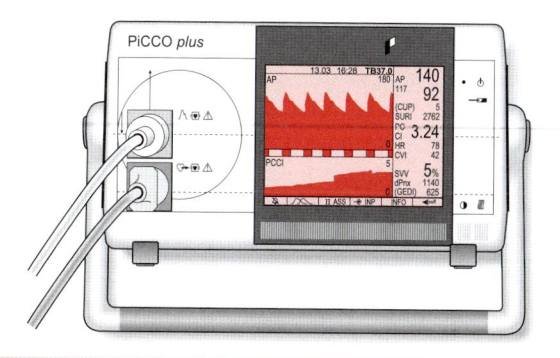

**Fig 3.10.1** PiCCO® system (Pulsion Medical Systems AG). Reproduced with kind permission from Pryor JA, Prasad SA. 2008 Physiotherapy for Respiratory and Cardiac Problems, 4th Edn. Edinburgh, UK: Churchill Livingstone.

parameters for arterial BP, heart rate, cardiac output, global end-diastolic blood pressure, intrathoracic blood volume index, cardiac function index, global ejection fraction, stroke volume, stroke volume variation and systemic vascular resistance.

### FINDINGS

All of the above invasive cardiac monitoring systems indicate the function of the heart and can assist in the assessment of the whole cardiovascular system. Changes in the cardiac function will assist the medical and physiotherapy team in assessing the response to intervention and guide future treatment. For example, if a patient has a large change in cardiac output during manual hyperinflation, this will aid future decisions on whether to repeat treatment or choose an alternative modality.

For implications of arterial blood pressure, see 3.5 Blood pressure; for CVP, see 3.11 Central venous pressure.

Pulmonary artery pressure and PiCCO®. Pulmonary artery pressure will increase in poor left ventricular function, fluid overload (hypervolaemia) and mitral valve disease. However, low measurements will be seen in hypovolaemia. This information is important to physiotherapists as hypervolaemia may be seen in conjunction with pulmonary oedema, whereas hypovolaemia may cause drying of secretions making them harder for the patient to expectorate. Also, hyper- or hypovolaemic patients will react differently to rehabilitation because of the extra demands placed on the heart and vascular system.

### DOCUMENTATION

Arterial BP (where available) is recorded as part of the cardiovascular section of a system-based assessment. It may also be necessary to document non-invasive BP if grossly different as any reason for the difference (e.g. poor arterial BP trace). Any other forms of invasive cardiac monitoring may be recorded as required or as appropriate for the assessment being completed.

## 3.11 CENTRAL VENOUS PRESSURE (CVP)

### DEFINITION

CVP reflects the amount of blood returning to the heart (right ventricular filling or 'preload'). It is usually monitored via a catheter situated within the superior vena cava.

## 3.11 Central venous pressure (CVP)

### PURPOSE

CVP measurement may be used to guide fluid therapy. It is useful for the physiotherapist as it can help us to identify patients who are:

- overloaded with fluid and at risk of developing pulmonary oedema
- dehydrated and may have dry tenacious secretions
- at risk of cardiovascular instability during treatment.

### PROCEDURE

The catheter can be inserted via the subclavian, the internal jugular or the femoral veins. The catheter is connected to a manometer that sits level with the right atrium of the heart (Fig. 3.11.1). A central line trace and value is seen on the patient's monitor (this is often blue). Within critical care, continuous measurements are possible. Heart function is indirectly measured by CVP; therefore, in the critically unwell patient more specific invasive monitoring may be utilized (see 3.10 (Invasive) Cardiac monitoring).

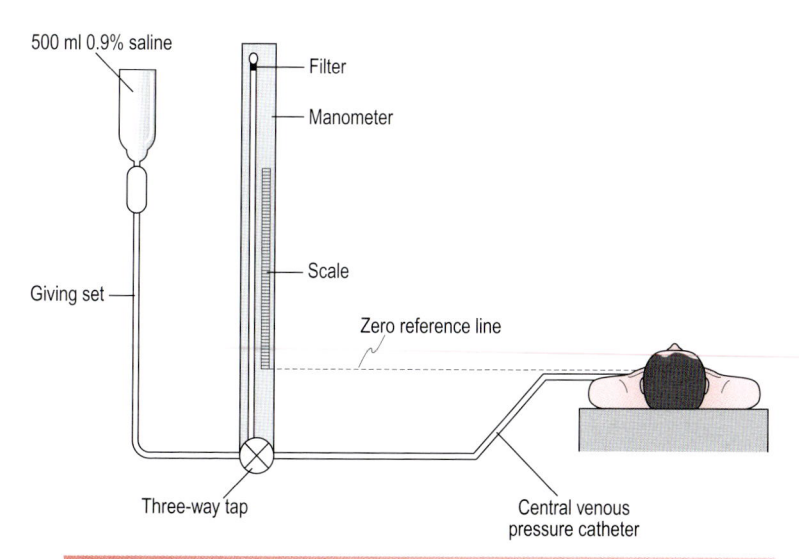

**Fig 3.11.1** Central venous pressure line set-up.
Reproduced with kind permission from Pryor JA, Prasad SA. 2008 Physiotherapy for Respiratory and Cardiac Problems, 4th Edn. Edinburgh, UK: Churchill Livingstone.

## ASSESSMENT TOOLS

### FINDINGS
- Normal CVP = 3–15 cmH$_2$O
- A high CVP may be associated with conditions that cause a rise in right atrial pressure such as heart failure, reduced right atrial compliance, tension pneumothorax, fluid overload or pulmonary hypertension.
- A low CVP may suggest hypovolaemia (reduced fluid) and gross vasodilatation of blood vessels (e.g. as in sepsis).
- Changes in CVP can provide information to the medical team on current fluid balance and also response to fluid loading.

### DOCUMENTATION
CVP should be documented under the CVS section of your assessment.

## 3.12 CEREBRAL PERFUSION PRESSURE (CPP)

### DEFINITION
Cerebral perfusion pressure (CPP) represents the pressure in the cerebral circulation that determines blood flow to the brain (perfusion). This value is calculated using the equation:

$$CPP = MAP - ICP$$

### PURPOSE
Monitoring CPP allows the team to identify whether the patient's brain has enough blood flow to prevent further damage and provide enough oxygen to the brain tissue. Physiotherapists must be aware of the CPP value as our treatment techniques may have an impact on both BP and ICP (intracerebral pressure) and therefore alter CPP – see 3.37 ICP.

### FINDINGS
The accepted value for CPP can be based on the individual, but commonly 50–90 mmHg is used. Persistently low pressures will cause brain ischaemia. High pressures may lead to bleeding and/or compression of brain tissue. Either situation could cause further brain damage.

If CPP is too high or too low, physiotherapy treatments (e.g. manual chest clearance, head-down positioning, suction or passive/active movements) may worsen the situation. They are likely to be contraindicated, or only used if considered essential to improve arterial oxygenation. If you do need to treat, determine whether the patient is stable enough and if there is any leeway if the BP should fall or the ICP should rise with treatment. Treatment decisions in this situation should be discussed with senior colleagues.

### DOCUMENTATION
The CPP value should be documented under the central nervous system (CNS) section of assessment and should be considered alongside MAP and ICP as well as the global clinical picture.

## 3.13 CHEST DRAINS

### DEFINITION
A chest (intercostal) drain is a tube inserted into the pleural space in order to drain air (pneumothorax) or fluid (pleural effusion, empyema, haemothorax or residual postoperative fluid) from the pleural space. The size of the tube can vary, from narrow bore (approximately 5 mm) to wide bore (approximately 1.5 cm). The tube leads away from the thorax to an underwater sealed unit which stops the drained fluid backtracking up the tube (Fig. 3.13.1). The drainage of fluid can be enhanced by the application of low-pressure suction. The tube will only be removed when it has stopped draining air or fluid.

### PURPOSE
Chest drains can be placed as part of a surgical procedure or to treat medical symptoms. It is important to observe the location and drainage of the chest drain as part of physiotherapy assessment as its presence may affect the patient's mobility and ability to expand the thorax. It is also important to notice whether the drain is blocked or not draining properly – this needs to be reported immediately.

### PROCEDURE
A simple look, listen and feel will tell you a lot:

- Look at where the drain enters the patient and the dressing around it. Do not take down the dressing, but look for oozing or leaks. Look at the tube and bottle forming the underwater seal and how the water level varies (Fig. 3.13.2).
- Listen to the patient – do they report any pain and how are they breathing?
- Feel the level of expansion of the chest.

## ASSESSMENT TOOLS

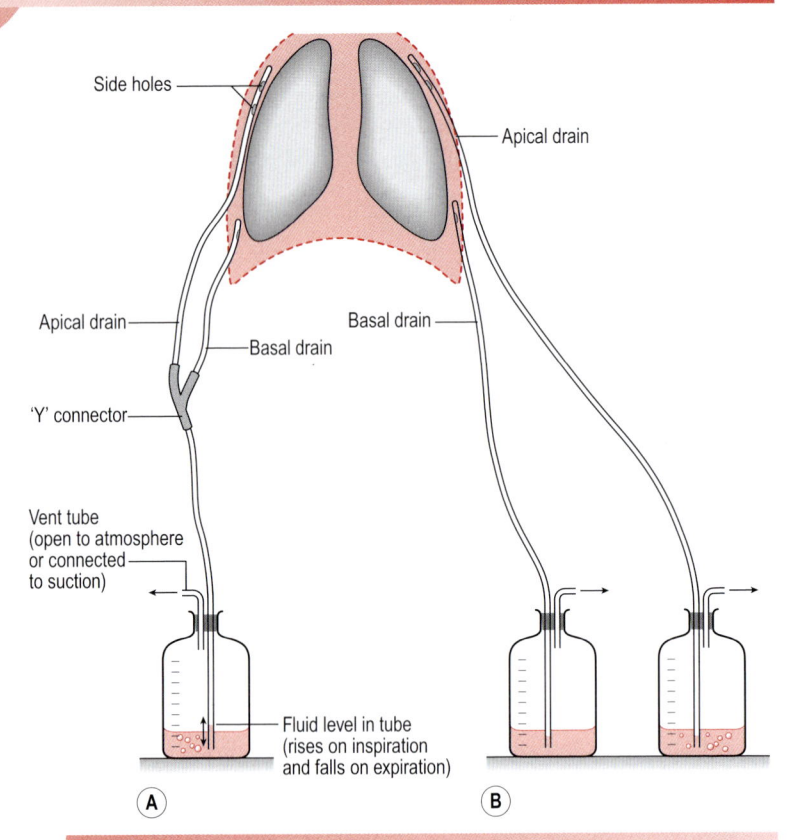

**Fig 3.13.1** Chest drain schematic. Underwater seal chest drainage. (A) single bottle system allowing use of one bottle via a 'Y' connector to drain fluid and air. (B) Two separate bottles enabling drainage of air from the apical drain and fluid from the basal drain Reproduced with kind permission from Pryor JA, Prasad SA. 2008 Physiotherapy for Respiratory and Cardiac Problems, 4th Edn. Edinburgh, UK: Churchill Livingstone.

### FINDINGS

The position of the chest drain will be assessed by the medical staff by chest radiograph.

Things to consider from a physiotherapy point of view:

- *'Swinging'*. The fluid in the tube should move during the respiratory cycle. If it is not swinging, check with the nursing staff. It could be that the tube is ready to come out, or that there is a problem with the tube. Check that the tube is not kinked or obviously blocked (by the patient sitting on it!). If not, discuss with the nursing or medical staff.

## 3.13 Chest drains

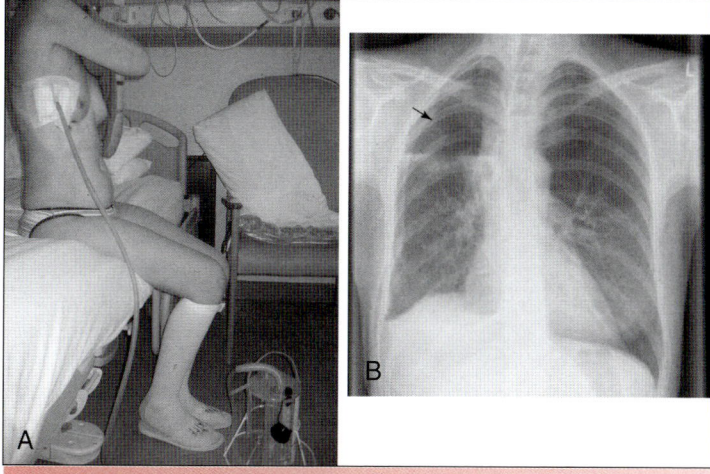

**Fig 3.13.2** Chest drain in situ post thoracotomy (A) and corresponding CXR (B). Note apical placement of drain (arrow).
Reproduced with kind permission from Harden B, Cross J, Broad M, et al. 2009 Respiratory Physiotherapy: An On-call Survival Guide, 2nd Edn. Edinburgh, UK: Churchill Livingstone.

- *'Bubbling'*. Occurs if there is an air leak and air bubbles are seen in the drainage bottle. It is important to note whether bubbling happens in part of the respiratory cycle or just on coughing as this gives an indication of the severity of the leak. So what should you do if it is bubbling? Is this a new occurrence or not? If this has not happened previously, you will need to highlight this to the team.
- *'Draining'*. The volume of fluid drained needs to be measured. How is the volume measured? The volume is measured in millilitres (ml) by looking at the graduated lines on the side of the chest drain bottle. Remember that the bottle is filled with approximately 500 ml of water to create a negative suction pressure in the pleural space; therefore, 500 ml needs to be subtracted from the total amount of drainage in the bottle to determine how much fluid had drained from the pleural space – this is generally allowed for by our nursing colleagues when they chart drainage.

Pain can be an issue, and the level should be recorded in relation to the respiratory cycle (the patient reports pain on deep breathing) or in relation to coughing. There should be adequate analgesia to allow the patient to move. You should also monitor the patient's arm movements, encouraging shoulder abduction (ordering a drink or waving movement), medial rotation (can they touch their back as if to do up a bra!) and lateral rotation (can the patient touch the back of the head to do their hair) and consider trunk movement, as this may be compromised.

> **Top tip!**
> A chest drain should always be below the level of the chest to prevent siphoning of the contents back into the chest cavity!
>
> Patients can mobilize with a chest drain in place and should be encouraged to do so – make sure the drain is held below the level of the chest!

### DOCUMENTATION
Document how the wound site appears, whether the drain is swinging or bubbling, and the volume of fluid drained during a certain time period (often 24 hours). Document any limited range of movement of shoulder joint or trunk.

## 3.14 CHEST IMAGING (INCLUDING CHEST X-RAYS)

### DEFINITION
Images of the thorax used to aid diagnosis include chest X-rays (CXR), computer tomography (CT) scans, magnetic resonance imaging (MRI), ultrasound imaging and nuclear medicine. Physiotherapists may seek information regarding the outcomes of scans but are usually only involved in interpretation of CXR images, so these will be the focus of this section.

### PURPOSE
Imaging is normally used by medical staff to aid diagnosis; however, physiotherapists often refer to this information to identify specific areas of loss of volume or collapse/consolidation that may respond to physiotherapy. Images may also be used as outcome measures for physiotherapy and may demonstrate improvements after sputum clearance or treatment to increase volume.

### Chest X-rays
Uses X-rays to generate an image of the thoracic anatomy. These are the mainstay of imaging in acute care. CXRs are normally taken from behind the patient (posterior to anterior (or PA) film) to reduce the shadow of the heart. In a ward or critical care environment they are frequently taken from the front (anterior to posterior (or AP) film) because of limitations caused by the position of the patient. Occasionally, films are taken from the side (a lateral film).

## 3.14 Chest imaging (including chest X-rays)

In modern radiology, images are stored and viewed using a picture archiving and communication system (PACS). This stores and retrieves images digitally and has the added benefit of allowing you to view any reports on the film.

### Computer tomography
This is an advanced form of X-ray scanning in which images are acquired from a 360° arc around the patient and reconstructed to give three-dimensional images of the study area. CT can be used to gain a much clearer picture of the structures within the chest. For example, prior to thoracic/lung surgery or to monitor disease progression as with cystic fibrosis (CF) or bronchiectasis. CT can also be used when pulmonary emboli are suspected (CTPA – CT pulmonary angiogram). CTs require a higher dose of ionizing radiation than a CXR.

### Magnetic resonance imaging
This uses strong magnetic fields to give detailed three-dimensional images (i.e. no ionizing radiation is used). MRI is rarely used in respiratory investigations and is much better for body parts with higher water content (e.g. joints) as this technology relies on magnetic fields exciting water molecules to produce an image.

### Ultrasound imaging
High-frequency sound waves are converted into an image using a probe over a localized area. This imaging process relies on a fluid medium to transmit the sound waves; therefore, it can be very useful to image the heart, effusions or other collections of fluid in the pleural space. Sometimes an ultrasound is used to identify where an effusion is and to mark a place on the skin to guide the doctors on where it should be drained.

### Nuclear medicine
This field of medicine uses a variety of radioactive isotopes with short half-lives, whose movement through the body can be detected. This can give information about physiological processes, for example ventilation/perfusion (V/Q) scans, although CTPA scans are more commonly used in preference.

### PROCEDURE
The procedures are performed by trained specialists, either medical staff or radiographers. A few specialist physiotherapists are involved in these procedures in both image acquisition and ordering imaging.

**70** ASSESSMENT TOOLS

### FINDINGS

The key to interpreting CXRs successfully is to take a systematic approach, otherwise you will miss something! Remember – do not view them in isolation. They are a useful diagnostic tool but do not give the whole story. Interpret the radiological evidence with the other clinical signs from your assessment and the patient's history. Does the CXR match the clinical picture? Think about surface and the internal anatomy of the chest. Remember that this is a two-dimensional projection of a three-dimensional structure.

It is accepted practice that you view the image as if the patient were standing in front of you, so the right side of the image is the left side of the patient. To save confusion, the radiographers label the image with an 'L' or 'R' (see Fig. 3.14.1, which shows a PA

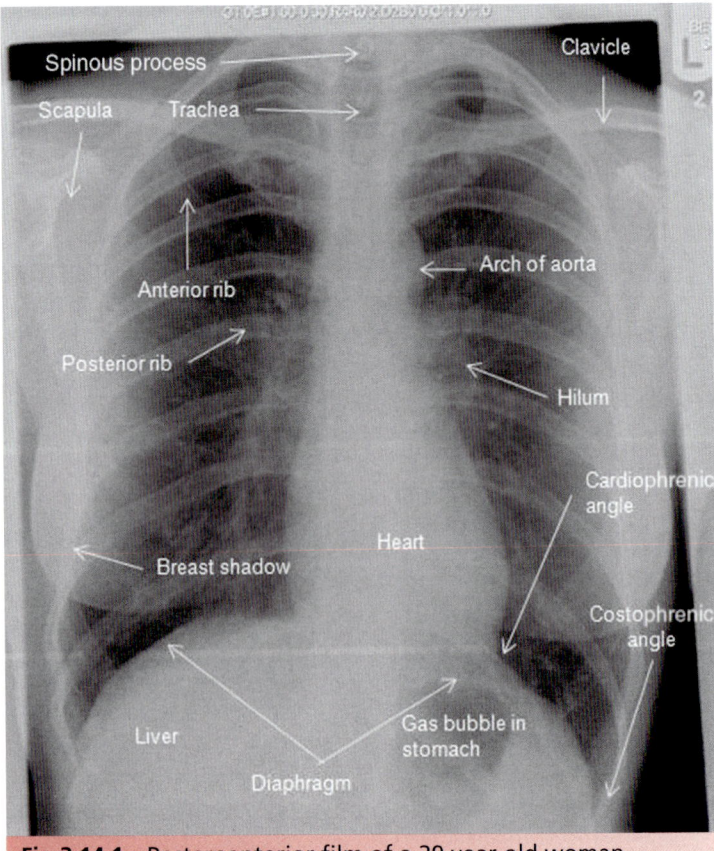

**Fig 3.14.1** Posteroanterior film of a 29 year old woman.

## 3.14 Chest imaging (including chest X-rays)

film of a healthy 29 year old woman with some of the anatomical structures annotated). Note that the white areas represent densities (e.g. the heart) whereas the blacker areas represent less dense areas (air shows as black). Table 3.14.1 highlights some simple questions to consider when reviewing a CXR.

In Fig. 3.14.2, the same CXR of the 29 year old woman is shown. It has been marked for ease of interpretation using the system for interpretation of CXRs summarized in Table 3.14.2. Use the suggested points while looking at the radiograph in Fig. 3.14.2. This is just one system that can be used to go through CXRs – the key is to use the same system every time so that you do not miss anything out!

It is particularly important for the physiotherapist to be able to identify loss of volume and consolidation as these may suggest the need for intervention. It is also important to be aware of a pneumothorax as this may be a contraindication to treatment. Pulmonary oedema and emphysema are also important; for further details, see Further reading.

| Table 3.14.1 | Questions to consider when reviewing a CXR |
|---|---|
| Who? | Who is the film of? A simple question but it is all too easy to look at the film of the wrong patient! |
| What? | What part of the body was radiographed? With PACS systems it is easy to bring up an image from another part of the body |
| When? | When was the film taken? You can look at an old film and wonder why the patient looks so well! It is also good to compare previous images with the most recent film to look for changes |
| Where? | Where was the film taken? A film taken on the ward will not be of the same quality as one taken in the department. Departmental films are taken with the shoulders protracted, thus keeping the scapula away from the lung fields |
| Why? | Why was the film taken in the first place? There is always a good clinical reason |
| How? | How was the film taken? AP vs PA. With an AP film the heart shadow is larger |

AP, anteroposterior; PA, posteroanterior.

# 72 ASSESSMENT TOOLS

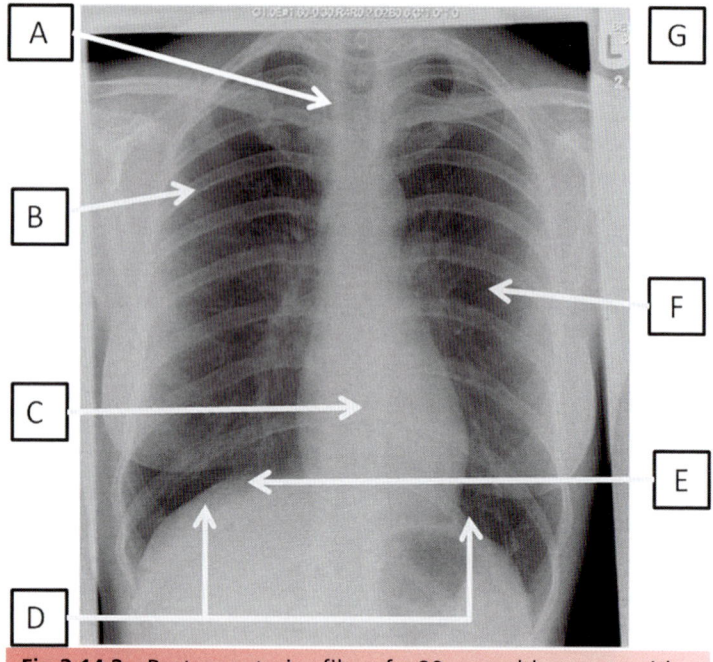

**Fig 3.14.2** Posteroanterior film of a 29 year old woman with CXR analysis markers - see Table 3.14.2.

**Table 3.14.2  A system for interpretation of CXR**

| | | |
|---|---|---|
| A | Alignment and A quick look! | Is there anything obviously wrong? Is it a straight film or rotated? If the patient was not straight at the time of the radiograph, the positions of the structures will appear to have moved. To assess this, look at the proximal ends of the clavicles – they should be an equal distance from the spinous processes. If they are not, the side with the bigger gap is the side it is rotated towards |
| B | Bones | Are they all there or are there bits that should not be there at all? Look for fractures, and not just of the ribs. In trauma patients these are frequently not picked up until much later on and it may be that you are the first person to notice it. There are no fractures in Fig. 3.14.2 |

## Table 3.14.2  A system for interpretation of CXR—cont'd

| | | |
|---|---|---|
| C | Cardiac | Look at the heart size and borders. The heart should be one-third of the diameter of the chest, with more on the left side than the right. The heart borders or lines around the heart should be smooth. There should also be a sharp angle seen between the heart borders and the diaphragm. These are known as cardiophrenic angles |
| D | Diaphragm | Can you see both of them clearly? The costophrenic angles between the ribs and the diaphragm should be clear and sharp. If not, there may be some fluid in the pleural space. Note that the right hemidiaphragm is always higher than the left hemidiaphragm owing to the position of the liver under the right lung |
| E | Expansion and Extrathoracic structures | Expansion is a reflection on the volume of air in the lungs. The normal level of expansion is to the 10th rib at the mid-clavicular point posteriorly or the 6th rib anteriorly. Underexpansion may mean poor lung volumes; overexpansion may be related to other pathologies, such as emphysema. Extrathoracic structures should be looked at for obvious changes or warning signs such as subcutaneous emphysema (air in the soft-tissue structures) |
| F | Fields | The lung fields are as a result of the vascular structures within the lung. As such, in an upright film there are more lung markings at the base than at the apex. These should extend to the edge of the chest wall. In pathological states, you should look for increased shadowing, decreased tissue density or absence of lung markings. You will need to be able to differentiate between collapse, consolidation, and air/fluid within the lung and outside the lung. In general, if there are areas of lung which have collapsed, the surrounding structures will shift towards that area; if there is consolidation, there will be an increase in the shadowing or 'whiteness' but with no shifting of structures |
| G | Gadgets | There may be a variety of drips, drains, tubes, lines, wires, orthopaedic fixtures and fittings, prosthetic valves, pacemakers. There are none in Fig. 3.14.2 |

## DOCUMENTATION

Identify any obvious abnormality compared with the normal presentation, and describe it in terms of how it differs from normal (e.g. there is an area of increased density in the right upper lobe).

## FURTHER READING

Corne, J., Pointon, K., 2009. Chest X-Ray Made Easy, 3rd edn. Churchill Livingstone, Edinburgh, UK.

## 3.15 CHEST X-RAY (See under 3.14 CHEST IMAGING – page 68)

## 3.16 CHEST WALL SHAPE

### DEFINITION

Identification of any variations of the skeletal structures of the thoracic cage, resulting in fixed or non-fixed changes that could affect respiration (e.g. the thoracic spine, ribs, sternum, clavicle and the associated joints).

### PURPOSE

To identify patients:

- at an increased risk of respiratory complications due to a restrictive breathing pattern (e.g. after surgery)
- who might benefit from exercise or mobilization to improve chest wall mobility
- with severe airway obstruction where the effect on lung mechanics could limit their ability to breathe diaphragmatically or take part in exercise.

### PROCEDURE

(Any significant deformity may already be recorded in the patient's notes.)

- Observe the patient with his or her top removed (if appropriate) from posterior, anterior and lateral aspects, and note any of the changes described in the findings below.

### FINDINGS

Variations in chest wall shape are shown in Fig. 3.16.1.

#### Restrictive changes

- Pes excavatum (funnel chest): the sternum is indented.
- Pes carinatum (pigeon chest): the sternum projects forwards.

## 3.16 Chest wall shape

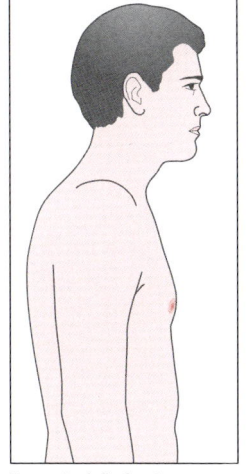

**Normal adult chest**

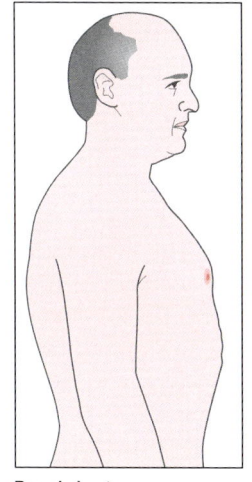

**Barrel chest**
Increased anteroposterior diameter

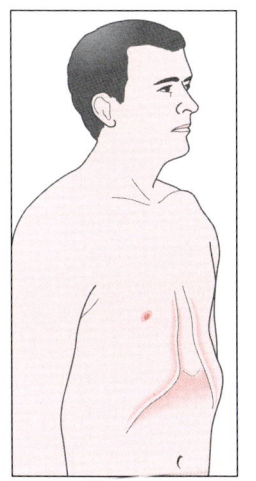

**Pigeon chest**
Anteriorly displaced sternum

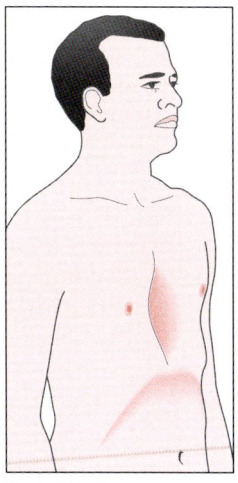

**Funnel chest**
Depressed lower sternum

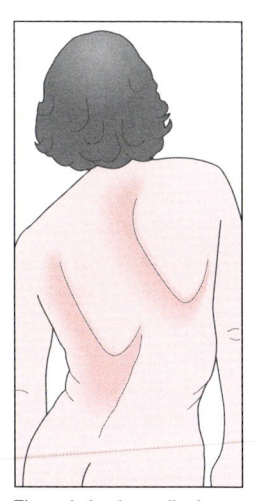

**Thoracic kyphoscoliosis**
Raised shoulder and scapula, thoracic convexity, and flared interspaces

**Fig 3.16.1** Chest wall shape.
Reproduced with kind permission from Lippincott, Williams and Wilkins 2004. Breath Sounds made Incredibly Easy. Springhouse Publishing Co.

- Scoliosis: the thoracic spine is curved laterally and rotated.
- Kyphosis: the thoracic spine is curved anteroposteriorly.
- Stiff, immobile ribs due to osteoarthritis, osteoporosis or previous rib fractures.
- Thoracoplasty – rib resection.

This can result in a reduced inspiratory capacity (inspiratory reserve) and predispose to 'low lung volumes', causing a restrictive pattern. This may result in a reduction in maximum voluntary ventilation, which in turn will lower potential exercise tolerance. These deformities may also increase the work of breathing.

These factors predispose the patient to atelectasis and possibly respiratory failure and fatigue (particularly if the patient is facing additional respiratory compromise, such as pneumonia or because of abdominal or thoracic surgery).

### Obstructive changes

Severe airway obstruction (e.g. severe COPD or CF) can lead to gas trapping and hyperinflated lungs that give rise to a barrel chest appearance. The chest appears deeper from front to back than normal and becomes more rounded. This is because the ribs are permanently elevated, even during expiration. Since the patient cannot lift the ribs very much further on inspiration (loss of bucket handle mechanism), they use their neck muscles to lift the clavicle and the whole thoracic cage in order to breathe in. They will have elevated clavicles and scapulae and a protracted shoulder girdle as a result of needing to use accessory muscles of inspiration.

Severe mechanical changes associated with obstruction will result in a flattened diaphragm that cannot descend much further. Therefore, teaching the patient diaphragmatic breathing would be inappropriate. Patients may need to fix their arms in front of the thorax in order to use their serratus anterior and pectoral muscles to help lift the thorax forwards in order to inspire, e.g. forward lean sitting.

#### Top tip!
These patients are working at a mechanical disadvantage. Therefore, when they are unwell, they have a limited respiratory reserve and so may deteriorate very quickly. They should be considered as at high risk of deterioration!

### DOCUMENTATION
State any observed variation in chest wall shape using above terminology under observation.

## 3.17 (DIGITAL) CLUBBING

### DEFINITION
Digital clubbing might be a sign of underlying or chronic lung disease. It is a deformity of the nail bed of fingers and toes associated primarily with cardiac, gastrointestinal or respiratory disease.

### PURPOSE
To identify patients with underlying respiratory or cardiac disease with significant hypoxia. The exact mechanism of developing clubbing is unclear; however, it is thought to be as a result of capillary proliferation. Digital clubbing usually occurs as a result of respiratory, cardiac or gut disease and occasionally can occur with no underlying pathology (Table 3.17.1).

### PROCEDURE
An examination of the hands and nail beds will identify clubbing.

### FINDINGS
Figure 3.17.1 demonstrates digital clubbing of a 24 year old man with CF compared with the finger of the author. Note the bulbous end of the patient's finger and loss of the acute angle in the nail bed.

### DOCUMENTATION
Note the presence of clubbing within the observations section of your assessment.

Table 3.17.1 Some causes of digital clubbing

| Respiratory | Cardiac | Gut | Other |
| --- | --- | --- | --- |
| Primary lung cancer<br>Lung abscess<br>Bronchiectasis and cystic fibrosis<br>Fibrotic lung disease | Infective endocarditis<br>Chronic cardiac failure<br>Congenital heart disease | Ulcerative colitis<br>Crohn's disease<br>Liver cirrhosis | Acromegaly<br>Hereditary |

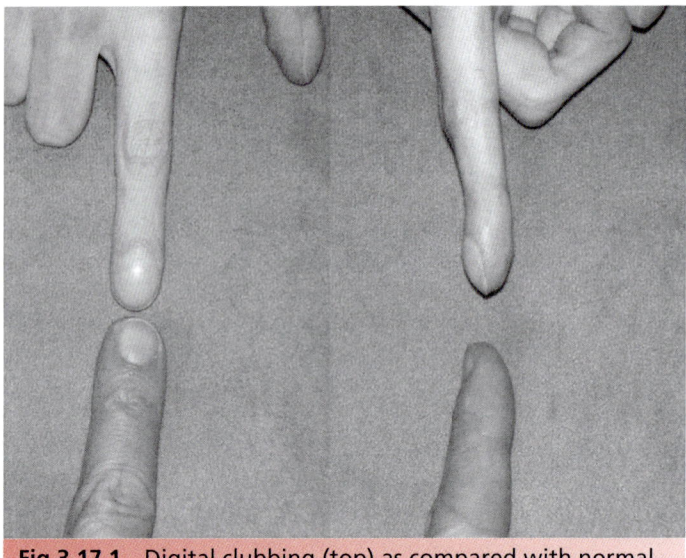

**Fig 3.17.1** Digital clubbing (top) as compared with normal.

## 3.18 CONSENT

### DEFINITION
The provision of approval or assent, particularly and especially after thoughtful consideration (Oxford English Dictionary). Remember that, for an adult, it is only the person themselves or a designated person (advocate) in the absence of the individual's capacity who can consent for treatment.

### PURPOSE
To allow a patient to consider relevant information to decide whether they want to be assessed or treated. If we treat without consent we could be accused of battery/assault. Some of our patients will not be able to consent; this may be because they are unconscious, are not able to communicate or lack capacity. In this instance, we are able to treat in their best interests.

### DOCUMENTATION
All consent issues and how consent is obtained should be documented clearly at the start of any new intervention or treatment; some examples of how this may be done include:

- patient nodded/mouthed/verbally consented to assessment and treatment

- patient advocate consented to assessment and treatment
- patient unable to consent; therefore, assess and treat in best interests.

It is not appropriate to use abbreviations such as 'VCG' (verbal consent given) or ticks to document consent as this is inappropriate use of abbreviations and ticks do not give any indication as to how consent was obtained.

## 3.19 COUGH ASSESSMENT

### DEFINITION
Assessment of the factors affecting cough effectiveness and/or any problems associated with coughing (e.g. weakness, bronchospasm).

### PURPOSE
- To determine whether cough is sufficient to maintain effective sputum clearance and identify factors adversely affecting cough effectiveness. Used to identify the most appropriate clearance intervention(s).
- To identify situations of excessive non-productive coughing that may respond to cough suppression (e.g. breathing control practice to reduce coughing).
- To identify problems associated with coughing that may be affecting the patient's health or quality of life.

### PROCEDURE
#### Cough effectiveness
If your patient has signs/symptoms of sputum retention (e.g. crackles) you need to assess their ability to cough (directed cough):

- sit the patient up/forward and ask them to take a deep breath in first and then to cough as hard as they can.

#### Cough suppression
If the patient complains of frequent coughing but does not produce any sputum and there are no signs of sputum retention, assess their breathing pattern to determine whether there are any signs of hyperventilation, anxiety or excessive mouth breathing. The patient may benefit from breathing control or relaxation and practising cough suppression.

#### Chronic cough
Carry out subjective questioning to identify any problems associated with frequent coughing such as fatigue, anxiety, embarrassment, social situations in which coughing is a problem, lack of

sleep, abdominal muscle strain, retching, fainting, or coughing fits which are difficult to control. Of note is that stress incontinence is common in chronic coughers.

- Use a questionnaire such as the Leicester cough questionnaire (LOC) in order to explore or quantify this further.

## FINDINGS

Potential factors affecting cough effectiveness:

- Can the patient take a deep breath in?
- Any inspiratory muscle weakness?
- Chest wall deformity or lack of mobility?
- Did you hear the glottis close, then open suddenly at the beginning of cough (the harsh sound that characterizes a cough) or did it sound more like a forced expiratory manoeuvre?
- Any pain that might be affecting cough? If so, consider pain control, or supported coughing if there is a wound or incision.
- Any wheezing? Patient may have airway obstruction affecting expiration – do they need bronchodilators?
- Does the patient have a condition which might cause weakness of the expiratory muscles? If so, could this respond to strengthening exercises or does the patient need some support such as manually assisted cough or the cough assist machine?
- Peak cough flow. The peak expiratory flow rate during cough gives an overall evaluation of cough efficiency; values below 160–270 l/min suggest poor airway clearance. A value of less than 160 l/min is not sufficient to clear secretions independently. It can be measured by coughing into a peak flow meter.
- Is the patient's airway at risk? (Loss of bulbar function; see 3.60 Swallow assessment.)
- Is the patient unable to cough in response to direction? Are there any neurological reasons for inhibited cough reflex or lack of sensitivity in the airways? Has the patient lost other protective reflexes such as the gag reflex, swallow reflex or the expiratory reflex? These reflexes are controlled by the medulla oblongata and are referred to collectively as 'bulbar function'.

### Top tip!
A problem with bulbar function may need urgent attention such as the recovery position, airway insertion or suction, so highlight to senior immediately.

## DOCUMENTATION

Record observations and the patient's response to any attempted intervention.

## FURTHER READING

Morice, A.H., Fontana, G.A., Belvisi, M.G., et al, 2007. ERS guidelines on the assessment of cough. Eur. Respir. J. 29, 1256–76.

University Hospitals of Leicester NHS Trust, 2001. Leicester Cough Questionnaire. Glenfield Hospital, Leicester, UK.

## 3.20 CYANOSIS

### DEFINITION

A bluish discoloration of the skin and/or the mucous membranes that is caused by lack of oxygen in the blood and local tissues:

- Central cyanosis appears around the mouth, tongue and lips.
- Peripheral cyanosis: only the peripheries are affected (especially fingers, fingernails, toes and toenails).

### PURPOSE

Central cyanosis may indicate significant respiratory or cardiac failure, which is potentially life-threatening, requiring immediate respiratory or circulatory support (see Findings below).

### PROCEDURE

Cyanosis can be observed directly through observation of the lips, tongue and fingers in good light.

### FINDINGS

- Cyanosis of recent onset should be immediately reported to the medical team.
- Cyanosis shows best on those with good levels of Hb. It is less visible in patients with anaemia.
- Cyanosis is usually only visible when 5 g Hb per 100 ml blood is deoxygenated. For most people in an acute situation, this would suggest a severe lack of oxygen and the need for immediate intervention (e.g. airway management, CPR, ventilation).
- People with severe chronic respiratory disease are more likely to show signs of cyanosis (at higher $S_pO_2$) because they may have more Hb (because of polycythaemia). Additionally, their oxygen content may actually be acceptable despite low $S_pO_2$; this is the result of increased Hb, which enables more oxygen to be carried, so it is important to find out whether this is 'usual' for them before responding.
- Note that cyanosis is more difficult to see in Afro-Caribbean and Asian patients because of darker skin tone.

## 82 ASSESSMENT TOOLS

### DOCUMENTATION

Record date and time, whether cyanosis is central and/or peripheral, on room air or oxygen therapy, the method of oxygen delivery and the percentage of any oxygen given.

## 3.21 DERMATOMES

### DEFINITION

A dermatome is an area of skin with sensory innervation by one main spinal nerve root (Fig. 3.21.1).

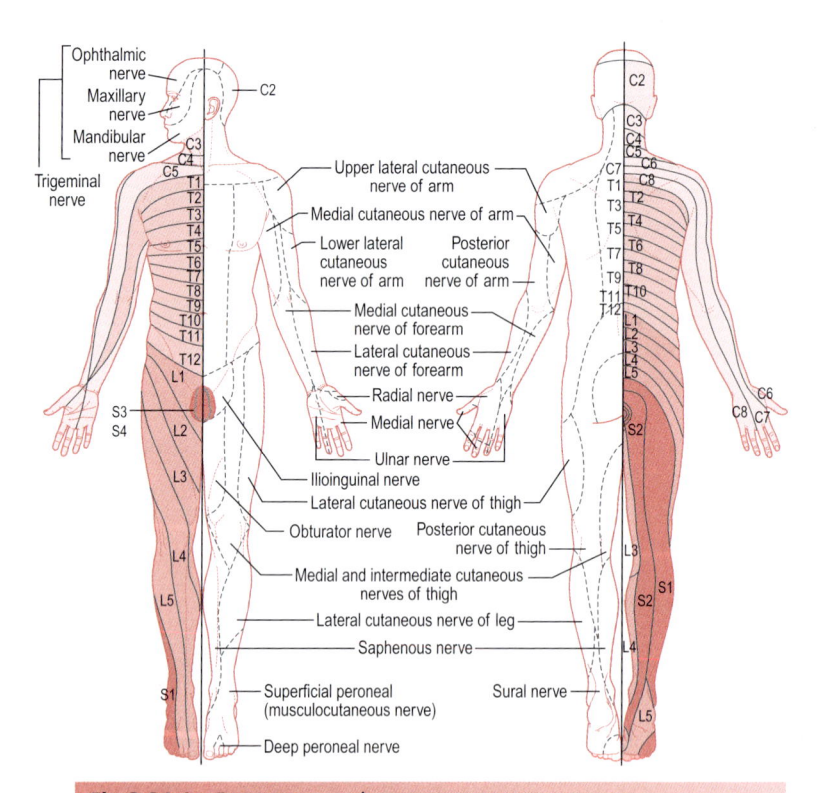

**Fig 3.21.1** Dermatome chart. n., nerve.
Reproduced with kind permission from Crossman AR, Neary D. 2002 Neuroanatomy: An Illustrated Colour Text, 2nd Edn. Edinburgh, UK: Churchill Livingstone.

## 3.21 Dermatomes

### PURPOSE

Knowing which nerve supplies an area of skin can be used to ascertain the level of injury or deficit. It should be noted that there is some overlap between dermatomes. Dermatome assessment is often carried out alongside assessment of myotomes and muscle charting (see 3.42 Myotomes and 3.41 Muscle charting).

Dermatomes can also be used to assess the level of analgesia, e.g. with an epidural.

### PROCEDURE

- Make sure any clothing that may restrict the assessment is removed (remember to maintain dignity of the patient).
- Using your hand, or a cotton wool ball, touch an area of skin that is unaffected to make sure the patient can feel this sensation.
- Ask the patient to close his or her eyes.
- Working from the top of the body down, stroke over different dermatomes and ask the patient to report changes in sensation. Make sure to compare left and right as deficits may be unilateral!

For the assessment of analgesia via epidural block, an ice pack rather than cotton wool is commonly used to assess the level at which the block is working.

Light touch and pinprick can also be assessed for differentiation between sensations (i.e. sharp and dull). This is commonly used in neurological assessment.

### FINDINGS

If an area is not innervated (e.g. no sensation) it may need to be protected from damage caused by lack of pain/temperature receptors.

It may be necessary to re-chart dermatomes on several occasions to assess improvement or deterioration in the level of sensation. This is particularly relevant in the management of early spinal injury in which 'spinal shock' (i.e. inflammatory response in the spinal cord) may cause a higher level of deficit than the original injury level. This needs to be closely monitored.

### DOCUMENTATION

Document at which level the patient can detect altered sensation (and which sensation you tested, e.g. sharp/dull/light touch) as per the dermatome chart (Fig. 3.21.1), e.g. 'Sensation to light touch present above T6 level'.

## FURTHER READING

Day, R., Fox, J., Paul-Taylor, G., 2009. Neuro-musculoskeletal Clinical Testing: A Clinician's Guide. Churchill Livingstone, Edinburgh, UK.

## 3.22 DRUGS

### DEFINITION

Physiotherapy assessment should include a list of the medications the patient is currently taking, how frequently they are taken and their drug history (DH) if appropriate.

### PURPOSE

A clear understanding of the medication a patient is taking is invaluable, as this may highlight additional points from the patient's past medical history that have not been identified. Sometimes, we need to ensure that patients have taken medications prior to physiotherapy treatment (e.g. pain relief or bronchodilators), whereas on other occasions certain medication may contraindicate physiotherapy treatments (e.g. patients on long-term steroids may not be able to tolerate chest wall percussion). Physiotherapists also need to be aware of possible side-effects of some medications in order to report any observations to the medical team. Remember that certain drugs can limit the interventions a therapist can use; therefore, a working knowledge of common drugs is important.

### PROCEDURE

There are a number of sources to obtain a DH. Most of this will come from the notes, drug charts, letters or a discussion with patients or family. Most physiotherapists are not involved in the prescription of drugs.

### FINDINGS

Tables 3.22.1–3.22.6 display some of the common classifications of medications patients may take. This is by no means comprehensive, and the reader is directed to other sources (such as a BNF (British National Formulary)) for more comprehensive information. Note that, if you come across a drug that is unfamiliar to you, you should ensure that you have an understanding of both what it is intended to treat and the implications for physiotherapy. The pharmacy team are an excellent resource if you cannot find what a drug is or why it is being used.

### Table 3.22.1 Common respiratory medications

| | Key drugs | Implication for physiotherapy |
|---|---|---|
| **Oxygen** | Oxygen should be viewed as a drug and as such be prescribed | High-dose oxygen in normal individuals over time can cause airway irritation (note that any patient who requires high-dose oxygen is very ill). There is a small population of patients with COPD who rely on hypoxic drive, and if given too much oxygen will stop breathing. However, treatment should not be denied to patients who will benefit from this vital treatment. Physiotherapists should monitor saturation levels during treatment, particularly movement and exercise. It may be acceptable to increase or decrease oxygen flow in certain situations – check with your supervisor regarding your local policy |
| **Bronchodilators** (see examples below): may be delivered by inhaler or nebulizer | | May need to be taken prior to chest clearance procedures or before exercise if the patient is 'tight' or 'wheezy'. Can be used to relieve breathlessness in an emergency. Check inhaler technique |
| $\beta_2$-agonist | Salbutamol, terbutaline (short acting) Salmeterol (Serevent), formoterol (Oxis) (long acting) | Can cause increased heart rate and tremors |

*(Continued)*

### Table 3.22.1 Common respiratory medications—cont'd

| | Key drugs | Implication for physiotherapy |
|---|---|---|
| Anticholinergic | Ipratropium bromide (Atrovent) (short acting) Tiotropium (long acting) | Can cause a dry mouth, which may make airway clearance more difficult |
| Xanthines (bronchodilators with some anti-inflammatory effect) | Theophylline Aminophylline Phyllocontin | Can cause increased heart rate |
| **Steroids** (inhaled); steroids may also be oral (see Table 3.22.6) | Beclometasone Fluticasone Budesonide | High-dose inhaled steroids have been associated with oral fungal infections. Encourage the patient to rinse their mouth after taking the drug |
| **Mucolytics** | Carbocystine Dornase Alfa (DNAse) Hypertonic saline | Reduces viscosity of secretions and aids airway clearance Carbocystine can cause GI bleeding Hypertonic saline can increase bronchospasm |

COPD, chronic obstructive pulmonary disease; GI, gastrointestinal.

### Table 3.22.2 Common cardiac medications

While these have been placed in broad categories, these agents can affect several aspects of cardiovascular physiology

| | Key drugs | Implication for physiotherapy |
|---|---|---|
| Inotropes (increase myocardial contractility) | Adrenaline (epinephrine) Noradrenaline (norepinephrine) Dopamine Dobutamine | Patients on inotropes are cardiovascularly unstable and need careful handling Monitor BP when treating |

### Table 3.22.2 Common cardiac medications—cont'd

| | | |
|---|---|---|
| Anti-arrhythmia drugs (also known as anti-arrhythmics) | Digoxin<br>Amiodarone<br>Adenosine | Be aware of an abnormal cardiac rhythm and seek help of senior staff if you are unsure whether the patient's clinical picture has changed |
| Beta (β)-blockers (reduce rate and strength of heart beat) | Atenolol<br>Labetolol | Patients may not be able to respond to increased workload; thus, you may not be able to use HR as a guide to exercise prescription. Consider using RPE as well |
| Vasodilators (increase coronary blood flow and control angina) | GTN | Caution if mobilizing the patient for the first time; if the patient complains of chest pain or breathlessness, seek senior support immediately! Ensure patients have GTN handy when exercising if it is prescribed |
| Calcium channel blockers (reduce myocardial contractility and BP) | Diltiazem<br>Lidoflaxine<br>Nifedipine<br>Verapamil | Caution if mobilizing for the first time as BP may drop – be aware of resting BP; you may need to repeat BP measurement during your intervention |
| Diuretics (increase urine production and can reduce BP) | Bendrofluazide<br>Furosemide<br>(Frusemide)<br>Bumetanide<br>Spironolactone | Increase the need to go to the toilet and can induce muscle cramps |
| Antihypertensive drugs | Captopril<br>Enalapril<br>Adalat | If a patient is on this medication, note that they have a history of increased blood pressure |

BP, blood pressure; GTN, glyceryl trinitrate; HR, heart rate; RPE, rating of perceived exertion.

# ASSESSMENT TOOLS

**Table 3.22.3 Common antibiotics**

|  | Key drugs | Implication for physiotherapy |
|---|---|---|
| Penicillins | Benzylpenicillin<br>Flucloxacillin<br>Amoxicillin | Any patient who is on antibiotics will have an infection and is likely to feel unwell. Side-effects of many of these antibiotics include nausea, vomiting and diarrhoea. It is important to adhere to infection control principles Note: some antibiotics (e.g. in CF/bronchiectasis) may be nebulized and should be taken after airway clearance techniques |
| Cephalosporins | Cefaclor<br>Cefetaxime | |
| Tetracyclines | Tetracycline<br>Doxycycline | |
| Aminoglycosides | Gentamicin | |

**Table 3.22.4 Analgesic medications**

The route of delivery is varied and can include inhaled, oral, intramuscular (i.m.) and intravenous (i.v.) routes and as a suppository. Care should be taken when mobilizing patients with epidurals in situ (in place) as they can become hypotensive (low BP) and may have altered motor control of their legs.

|  | Key drugs | Implication for physiotherapy |
|---|---|---|
| Paracetamol |  | Risk of liver toxicity, and is often contained in other preparations |
| NSAIDs | Ibuprofen<br>Voltarol | Can cause irritation of the gut and cause GI bleeding. Some asthmatic patients are allergic to this group of drugs |
| Opiates | Morphine<br>Diamorphine<br>Codeine | Can depress the respiratory drive if the dose is too high. Pinpoint pupils may indicate that the patient has had a large dose of opiates |

GI, gastrointestinal; NSAID, non-steroidal anti-inflammatory drug.

**Table 3.22.5 Intensive therapy unit drugs**

|  | Key drugs | Implication for physiotherapy |
|---|---|---|
| Sedation agents | Midazolam<br>Propofol<br>Fentanyl | The patient may vary from being awake and settled to not being able to respond to you |
| Paralysing agents | Vecuronium<br>Pancuronium<br>Atracurium | BE AWARE! The patient can make no muscular effort at all, so if removed from the ventilator the patient will stop breathing. As patients are paralysed, they will not be able to cough on suction |

**Table 3.22.6  Other common drugs**

|  | Key drugs | Implication for physiotherapy |
|---|---|---|
| Anti coagulants (blood thinners) | Heparin<br>Warfarin<br>Aspirin<br>Clexane | There is an increased risk of bleeding, so care needs to be taken and some procedures considered with extreme caution, e.g. nasopharyngeal suction. Check the patient's clotting screen! (see 3.6 Blood results) |
| Insulins | Actrapid<br>Humulin<br>Mixtard<br>Gliclazide | If your patient is on insulin, it is good practice to ensure that blood sugars are stable prior to mobilizing. If the patient's blood sugars are poorly controlled they may become unresponsive |
| Immunosuppressant | Cyclosporin | As the immune system is suppressed, this leaves the patient more open to contracting infections |
| Steroids (oral/i.v.) | Prednisolone<br>Dexamethasone<br>Hydrocortisone | Long-term use can lead to diabetes, osteoporosis and a degree of immunosuppression Take care with manual clearance techniques if affected |
| Anti-epileptics | Carbamazepine<br>Phenytoin<br>Valproate | Be aware that the patient may have a history of fitting |

The majority of physiotherapists are non-prescribing. When a drug is prescribed, the prescription will state the drug, the dose, the route (i.v., oral, etc.), the frequency (as required (prn) or at set intervals) and the duration of the course (how many days). The person prescribing the drug should clearly sign the chart and ideally leave contact details.

The route is important as this implies different severities of the disease and the care required. For example, drugs delivered via an infusion imply that the patient is unwell (hence the need for an intravenous line) and care should be taken over the line delivering the drug.

## ASSESSMENT TOOLS

### DOCUMENTATION

The medications a patient is taking should be marked in the DH of your assessment, and any cautions/contraindications to physiotherapy intervention arising from the patient's medications should be noted clearly.

### FURTHER READING

The BNF is updated regularly, so look for the latest version as a hard copy or go to http://bnf.org

## 3.23 EARLY WARNING SCORES (EWS)

### DEFINITION

Simple scoring systems based on physiological measurements to assist staff to recognize and respond to the acutely unwell patient in hospital. Parameters measured can include HR, BP, RR, $S_pO_2$ and AVPU.

### PURPOSE

There are a large number of different early warning score (EWS) systems that are used, but all take physiological parameters and put a score to them. These scores can then be used to grade the severity of illness, identifying patients who need preventative treatment or should be moved to a higher dependency area (Table 3.23.1). For the purpose of this section we will use the modified early warning score (MEWS). See 3.61 TPR for a completed TPR chart example.

### PROCEDURE

The normal observations are taken and then scored according to Table 3.23.1. The overall score is then calculated and action is taken based on the score recorded (see below).

### FINDINGS

The key point is to look for a change in the score. A MEWS score which has changed by 3 or more would merit some form of action.

- Low score (1–3): increased frequency of observations.
- Medium score (3–6): urgent call to the team caring for the patient for a review.
- High score (>6): emergency medical treatment.

Even if your patient does not meet the 'trigger' score for review but you are concerned about them, this does not mean you cannot seek additional review.

## 3.23 Early warning scores (EWS)

Table 3.23.1 The original modified early warning score

| | 3 | 2 | 1 | 0 | 1 | 2 | 3 |
|---|---|---|---|---|---|---|---|
| Systolic BP (mmHg) | <70 | 71–80 | 81–100 | 101–199 | | ≥200 | |
| Heart rate (beats per minute) | | <40 | 41–50 | 51–100 | 101–110 | 111–129 | ≥130 |
| Respiratory rate (breaths per minute) | | <9 | | 9–14 | 15–20 | 21–29 | ≥30 |
| Temperature (°C) | | <35 | | 35–38.4 | | ≥38.5 | |
| AVPU score | | | | Alert | Reacting to Voice | Reacting to Pain | Unresponsive |

Reproduced with kind permission from Subbe et al (2001).

## ASSESSMENT TOOLS

### DOCUMENTATION

A postoperative patient currently has a blood pressure of 82/60 (score 1), with a pulse of 135 (score 3), a RR of 24 (score 2), a temperature of 39°C (score 2). This would be documented as a MEWS score of 8 (i.e. requiring an urgent medical review).

### FURTHER READING

National Institute for Health and Clinical Excellence, 2007. Acutely Ill Patients in Hospital. Clinical Guideline 50. NICE, London, UK. Available at: www.nice.org.uk/Guidance/GC50

Subbe, C.P., Kruger, M., Rutherford, P., Gemmel, L., 2001. Validation of a modified early warning score in medical admissions. Q. J. Med. 94, 521–6.

## 3.24 ELECTROCARDIOGRAM (ECG)
### (See under 3.35 HEART RHYTHMS – page 109)

## 3.25 ELECTROLYTES (See under 3.6 BLOOD RESULTS – page 49)

## 3.26 END-TIDAL CARBON DIOXIDE (ETCO$_2$)

### DEFINITION

Non-invasive measurement of carbon dioxide levels by sampling the air at the end of expiration, which 'approximates' the partial pressure of carbon dioxide in arterial blood ($P_aCO_2$). The device may be attached to an endotracheal tube (ETT) (with intubated patients) or can be positioned at the nose or mouth to sample expired air with non-intubated patients. Machines may incorporate a capnograph (a device that measure $CO_2$; Fig. 3.26.1), which also displays the flow waveform on a screen and allows more accurate interpretation of the end-tidal carbon dioxide (ETCO$_2$) levels. The device also measures respiratory rate (RR) and gives a continuous measurement that may be used to detect slow or fast breathing (Fig. 3.26.2).

### PURPOSE

- The main use is as a monitor with ventilated patients on ITU to highlight any problems with the ventilator settings and set-up. Often used after intubation to ensure that the endotracheal tube is positioned correctly.

## 3.26 End-tidal carbon dioxide (ETCO$_2$)

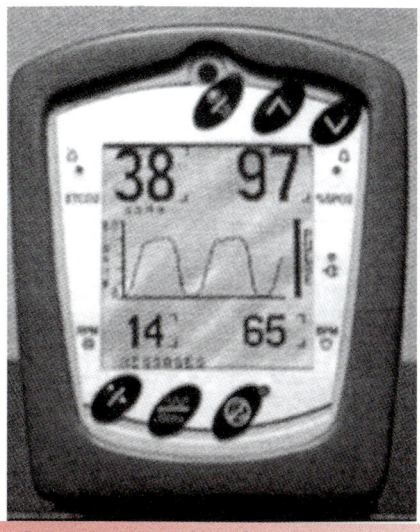

**Fig 3.26.1** Capnometry with self-ventilating patient.
Reproduced with kind permission from Al-Shaikh B, Stacey S. 2007 Essentials of Anaesthetic Equipment, 3rd Edn. Edinburgh, UK: Churchill Livingstone.

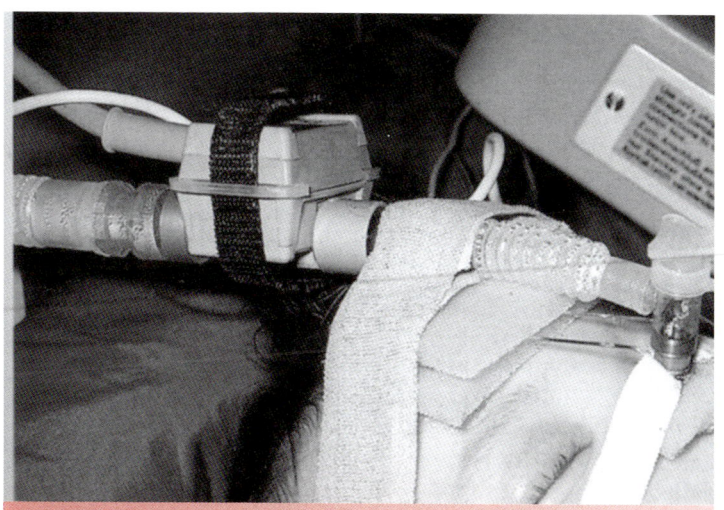

**Fig 3.26.2** Capnometry on ITU.
Reproduced with kind permission from Al-Shaikh B, Stacey S. 2007 Essentials of Anaesthetic Equipment, 3rd Edn. Edinburgh, UK: Churchill Livingstone.

- In self-ventilating patients, it can be used to detect and give feedback on lowered $CO_2$ levels for patients who are hyperventilating (overbreathing).

## PROCEDURE
- Measurement of $ETCO_2$ in ITU is normally a nursing procedure.
- Physiotherapists may use the following procedure to measure $ETCO_2$ when working with self-ventilating patients with dysfunctional breathing syndrome:
  - use a new sterile nasal prong for each patient
  - position (or ask patient to place) the probe in one nostril – near the end of the nose
  - encourage the patient to breathe normally and wait until $ETCO_2$ levels 'settle' and the RR is shown
  - this equipment is for single patient use; therefore, either clean and store for use again with the same patient or discard.

## FINDINGS
- Normal values for $ETCO_2$ are between 4.5 and 6 kPa, 35 and 45 mmHg, or 4% and 6% if measured as a percentage of the air.
- $ETCO_2$ is usually about 2–5 mmHg less than $P_aCO_2$, which gives a reasonable approximation of $P_aCO_2$; however, this close relationship is altered with:
  - ventilation/perfusion (V/Q) mismatch – common with respiratory disease
  - circulatory instability (e.g. pulmonary embolism, cardiac dysrhythmia)
  - unstable body temperature.
- With ventilated patients it is particularly important to consider the shape of the waveform trace when interpreting $ETCO_2$ measurements, as an abnormal tracing (that does not resemble Fig. 3.26.3) may be associated with inaccurate reflection of $P_aCO_2$.
- It is important to consider trends rather than one-off measurements, and to interpret the findings with caution, taking into account the other assessment findings as well.
- A trend towards increasing $ETCO_2$ (above 6 kPa or 45 mmHg) suggests hypoventilation (possibly related to secretion retention or exhaustion).
- A trend towards reducing $ETCO_2$ (below 4.5 kPa or 35 mmHg) may occur for a number of reasons with ventilated

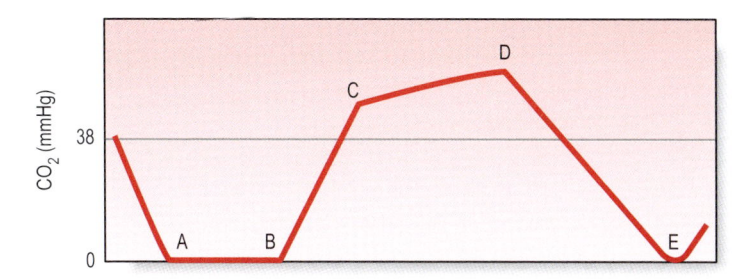

**Fig 3.26.3** Capnograph: normal waveform. Shows normal end-tidal carbon dioxide level. (A–B) Dead space ($CO_2$-free gas); (B–C) mixed dead space and alveolar gas; (C–D) mostly alveolar gas; (D) end-tidal $CO_2$; (D–E) inhaled gas ($CO_2$-free gas). Reproduced with kind permission from Pryor JA, Prasad SA. 2008 Physiotherapy for Respiratory and Cardiac Problems, 4th Edn. Edinburgh, UK: Churchill Livingstone.

patients (such as a leak in the cuff around the ETT, or ventilator disconnection), but with free-breathing patients it indicates hyperventilation (overbreathing).

### DOCUMENTATION

Record the position of the patient and $ETCO_2$ reading in kPa or mmHg depending on your local policy. Add any information about activity levels, inspired oxygen levels, any ventilatory support or any factors affecting the patient at the time of measurement.

## 3.27 EXERCISE (AEROBIC FITNESS) TESTING

### DEFINITION

Planned, controlled and supervised exercise protocols (usually involving walking, running, cycling or stepping) aimed at identifying maximum (or peak) aerobic exercise capacity and/or to observe physiological responses to specified exercise intensities.

### PURPOSE

- For exercise prescription, results may be used to calculate a safe and appropriate intensity for exercise training programmes such as pulmonary or cardiac rehabilitation.
- For an ambulatory oxygen assessment (compared with and without ambulatory oxygen).

- As a goal or target to help motivate patients.
- As an outcome measure to test the effects of treatments and interventions.
- Diagnosis and evaluation of disease.

## PROCEDURE

There are a number of validated exercise protocols – select the protocol that is most appropriate for the patient:

### Cardiopulmonary exercise test (CPET)

This is a laboratory-based treadmill or cycle ergometer test with a specific protocol and direct measurement of oxygen uptake until the maximum level ($VO_2$max) is achieved. It is commonly used for 'exercise stress tests' to aid diagnosis and management of cardiac patients. This test requires trained staff with current advanced life support certification, and equipment such as a gas analyser, ECG, blood pressure and lactate monitoring, and full resuscitation equipment including a defibrillator. The Bruce protocol is commonly used for the treadmill test (Fig. 3.27.1) - see Further reading.

### Field tests

These tests can be carried out in hospital and gym environments. They do not directly measure expired air, and do not monitor the patient as extensively as the cardiopulmonary exercise tests. (These tests do not measure $VO_2$max directly but they may be used to predict $VO_2$peak.) They are often more functional and better related to activities of daily living than a laboratory-based test.

Exercise tests may be classified under the following headings (e.g. the incremental shuttle walking test may be classified as an externally paced, incremental, maximal test).

### Externally paced or self-paced

- Externally paced tests usually use a pre-recorded signal that the patient has to keep pace with (e.g. shuttle walking tests, Chester step test; Fig. 3.27.2).
- Self-paced tests allow the patient to maintain the fastest speed that they can for the duration of the test, e.g. 6 or 12 minute walk test, 6 or 12 minute step test.

### Incremental or constant speed

- Incremental tests start at a slow pace and incorporate progressive 'stages' in which the speed is increased at specified levels (e.g. incremental shuttle walking test, Chester step test; Fig. 3.27.3).

## 3.27 Exercise (aerobic fitness) testing

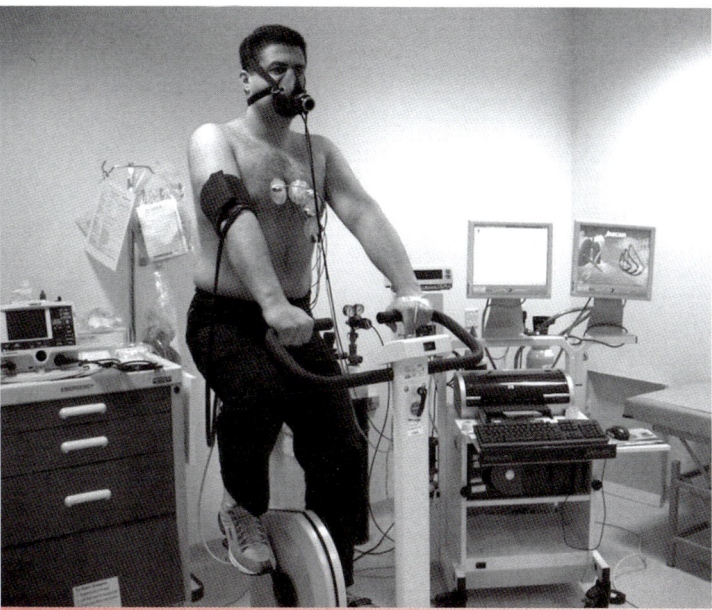

**Fig 3.27.1** Cardiopulmonary exercise test in the laboratory. Reproduced with kind permission from Albouaini K, Egred M, Alahmar A, et al. 2007 Cardiopulmonary exercise testing and its application. Postgraduate Medical Journal 83: 675–82.

- Constant speed tests can be used when testing endurance and for submaximal testing (e.g. endurance shuttle walking test).

*Maximal or submaximal:* Most tests are 'maximal' in that they require the patient to keep going until they cannot go any faster. They, therefore, aim to find the patient's 'peak' intensity of exercise. Submaximal tests, however, look at the patient's responses to a period of relatively low-intensity exercise that may then be used to 'predict' that person's peak intensity using a specified formula.

### Before an exercise test

- **Risk/safety assessment – health screening.**
  Ensure no contraindications – the following health checks should be made:
    - Recent infection: maximum exercise should not be undertaken if the patient has had any recent infection (within the past 2 weeks).
    - Cardiovascular risk: patients with a high risk of cardiovascular disease, recent heart attack or stroke (within 6 weeks)

**Fig 3.27.2** Shuttle walking test.

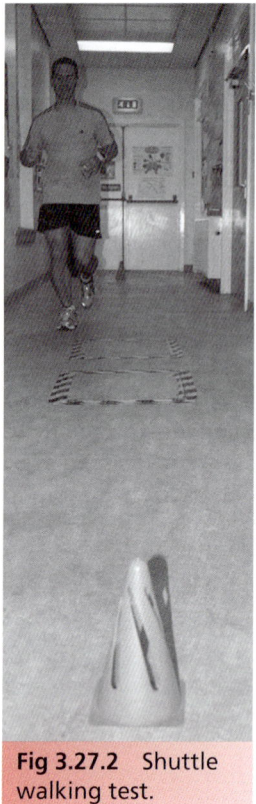

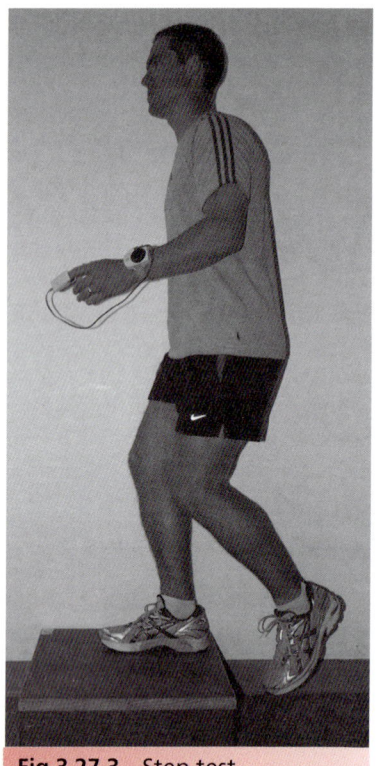

**Fig 3.27.3** Step test.

   should be referred to an appropriate medical practitioner for assessment prior to any exercise testing.
 – Blood pressure: resting BP should be between 60 and 90 mmHg (diastolic) and 100 and 140 mmHg (systolic) and be 'normal' for the patient; if not, further investigations should be carried out to ensure that the patient is safe to exercise.
 – Recent injury: any recent musculoskeletal injury (within 6 weeks) must be investigated and cleared prior to exercise testing.
 – Adverse symptoms: any pain, dizziness, fainting, incoordination, or any other symptoms or concerns should be investigated to ensure that the patient is safe to exercise.
 – Recent intensive exercise: people should not work maximally if they have carried out intensive exercise in the past 24 hours.

- Diabetes: ensure this is well controlled. For insulin-dependent diabetics, ensure that the timing of exercise is suitable and a sugary snack is available if needed. Discuss symptom recognition and response with the patient and ensure that you know how to respond if the patient becomes hypoglycaemic during exercise.
- **Check environmental factors:**
  - Floor must be dry and clear – any equipment, e.g. step or bike, must be tested for safety.
  - Check clothing for suitable shoes, ensure shoelaces are tied, secure any loose clothing that could cause the patient to trip.
  - Familiarize yourself with crash/first aid procedures and ensure you have access to a telephone, first aid box and also a crash team and crash trolley if working with high-risk patients.
  - The patient should not have eaten a meal or drunk any caffeine or alcohol for 2 hours prior to the test.
  - Record the temperature of the room and ensure that it is comfortable for exercise.
  - Ensure that drinking water is available.
  - Provide seating near to the test area in case the patient suddenly needs to rest.
  - Warn the patient to stop if they experience any pain, discomfort or dizziness and inform him/her of the risk of muscle aching (delayed-onset muscle soreness) for the following couple of days.

## Pre-test measurements

Take and record resting levels for the following as appropriate:

- HR
- BP
- RR
- breathlessness score (e.g. Borg)
- oxygen saturations ($S_pO_2$)
- any oxygen requirements.

## During the test

For each 'stage' of the test (or every 1–2 minutes):

- Note exercise achieved (e.g. protocol stage reached, number of steps, number of lengths).
- Monitor HR and $S_pO_2$ if using portable monitors (e.g. HR monitor, oximeter).
- Monitor carefully for any signs of dizziness, loss of coordination, pain or anxiety; stop the test and investigate if you observe these signs.

- Encourage and give feedback to the patient regarding his/her progress.
- Remind the patient that he/she can stop if needed (e.g. if any of the previously discussed symptoms arise).

## After the test
- Warm down for 5 minutes at a slower speed or allow the patient to sit and rest, as appropriate.
- Take post-test levels for the following as appropriate:
  - HR
  - BP
  - RR
  - breathlessness score (e.g. BORG)
  - $S_pO_2$
  - rating of perceived exertion (RPE) score.
- Identify any reasons for stopping, any limitations or symptoms experienced during the test.
- Offer the patient a drink of water.
- Ensure that the patient has returned to within five beats of resting HR and has no adverse symptoms before they leave the test area.
- Inform the patient of follow up – who to contact if they have any problems or pain following the test.

## FINDINGS
- Calculate $VO_2$peak. This is an estimate of the maximum oxygen uptake achieved when working at the highest stage or level of the test. It can be estimated by using the tables provided with the protocol or by using a standard formula for the type of exercise undertaken (see American College of Sports Medicine guidelines).
- Exercise intensity for further training can be prescribed at 50–85% of $VO_2$peak as appropriate.
- Use HR response and Borg breathless score or RPE to consider how close the patient came to his/her 'maximum' exercise capacity during the test (see 3.8 Breathlessness (dyspnoea) scales and 3.51 Rating of perceived exertion).
- Follow-up any problems, limitations or symptoms identified during the test with the appropriate practitioner.

## DOCUMENTATION
Record any pre-test health screen findings, safety warnings and patient consent, pre- and post-test measurements, type of test carried out, stage or level achieved, HR and $S_pO_2$ response for each stage, reasons for stopping and any symptoms or problems experienced, describe any warm-up or warm-down. Recovery time to resting HR should also be noted.

## FURTHER READING

American College of Sports Medicine, 2007. Physical Activity and Public Health Guidelines for Healthy Adults. ACSM, Indianapolis, IN.

American College of Sports Medicine, 2007. Physical Activity and Public Health Guidelines for Older Adults. ACSM, Indianapolis, IN.

Bruce, R., 1963. Bruce Protocol. Available at: http://www.brianmac.co.uk/bruce.htm

Sykes, K., 1998. Chester Step Test. Chester College of Higher Education, Chester, UK. Available at: http://www.topendsports.com/testing/history-sykes.htm.

University Hospitals of Leicester NHS Trust, Incremental shuttle walking test and endurance shuttle walking test. Available at: Pulmonary Rehabilitation Department, University Hospitals of Leicester NHS Trust, Glenfield Hospital, Groby Road, Leicester LE3 9QP, UK.

## 3.28 EXERCISE TOLERANCE

### DEFINITION

Exercise tolerance can be defined as an individual's capacity to exercise.

This could be:

- Self reported: the patient is asked how long he/she could continue with exercise before becoming fatigued (endurance).
- Measured: the maximum workload achieved during an exercise test (see 3.27 Exercise (aerobic fitness) testing).

### PURPOSE

Self-reported exercise tolerance gives a quick indication of any improvement or deterioration in the patient's condition over time and can be used to identify those patients in need of exercise interventions and/or social support. It can be taken into account when mobilizing patients or making decisions regarding suitability for discharge but is not as accurate or reliable as the results from a well-conducted exercise test.

### PROCEDURE

- Ask the patient to give a subjective assessment of his/her exercise tolerance, e.g. 'How far are you usually able to walk before becoming too tired to go any further?' or 'How many steps can you usually climb before becoming too tired to go any further?'
- Specify whether the distance walked is on the flat or includes hills.
- Exercise tolerance may vary according to any symptoms, time of day, and weather conditions so ask supplementary questions for further specificity.
- You may need to qualify this by suggesting a time period, e.g. 'over the past 2 weeks', and note whether this has been stable or getting better or worse recently.

# ASSESSMENT TOOLS

- Is the patient satisfied with this level of exercise tolerance or would he/she like to be able to do more?
- For some patients (e.g. those who are unable to walk) exercise tolerance may be based on the distance they can wheel themselves in their wheelchair, or their ability to transfer.
- It may be useful to estimate exercise tolerance from activities of daily living, e.g. are they able to wash themselves (face and hands, or all over body) or clean their teeth before becoming too tired to continue?
- Patients may also be asked to rate how hard an activity is by using the rating of perceived exertion scale (see 3.51 Rating of perceived exertion).

## FINDINGS

If the patient's exercise tolerance has been getting worse recently, this should be investigated further to identify possible causes such as deterioration in health status.

Patients with very poor exercise tolerance may be at higher risk of complications following surgery and may need more intensive rehabilitation prior to discharge.

## DOCUMENTATION

Record distance walked/number of steps climbed and time taken to walk a specified distance, if appropriate. Make a note of how the patient is/is not affected by weather conditions or any other factors. State whether this is less or more than when previously recorded if appropriate. You may find this recorded within the social history section of an initial database.

## 3.29 $FEV_1$/FVC (See under 3.40 LUNG VOLUMES AND LUNG FUNCTION TESTS – page 120)

## 3.30 FLOW VOLUME LOOPS (See under 3.40 LUNG VOLUMES AND LUNG FUNCTION TESTS – page 120)

## 3.31 FLUID BALANCE (INCLUDING URINE OUTPUT)

### DEFINITION

The running calculation of fluids that have been delivered minus those that have been excreted/drained from the body.

## 3.31 Fluid balance (including urine output)

### PURPOSE

In illness fluid balance is very important as patients who have lost lots of fluid are at risk of going into shock (a state of organ hypoperfusion) and therefore need to be monitored closely. Patients who have fluid overload may develop pulmonary oedema, which may lead to respiratory symptoms.

### PROCEDURE

In the ward setting, a fluid balance chart may be done over a 24 hour period (i.e. only a balance at the end of the day). Within critical care, there is a running hourly total. In both instances, this is completed by the nursing staff.

Fluid may be delivered orally, via a nasogastric (NG) tube or through an i.v. line. Fluid is normally lost through urine output and faeces. In the unwell patient fluid can additionally be lost from NG tubes and surgical drains. There are also insensible losses, including water vapour from the lungs and perspiration from the skin (these often increase in illness) – these cannot be recorded. See Fig. 3.31.1 for an example of a fluid balance chart.

### FINDINGS

Normal urine output is 0.5–1 ml/kg/hr in adults. In the unwell patient, a drop in urine output is often an early sign of deterioration and should be considered alongside the rest of your assessment.

Following surgery, drains are often used, and these are placed to drain excess fluid from a surgical site. This is often a slow drainage; therefore, if there is a large volume in the drain bag or if you note there is a large output you should seek senior help.

For specific information on chest drains, see 3.13 Chest drains.

- *Fluid loss/dehydration*: it is not uncommon for dehydration to be the result of too little fluid intake; remember that there are many patient groups that might not be able to drink independently, e.g. the grossly weak. Patients with diarrhoea and vomiting will have excessive fluid losses as will those following trauma or surgery – this can result in impairment of the body's electrolytes (see 3.6 Blood results) and also the acid–base balance (see 3.1 Arterial blood gases). Note that dehydration can cause sputum to become more viscous.
- *Fluid overload*: too much fluid is not uncommon in heart failure and kidney failure. It can also be the result of excessive sodium absorption. This can be due to too much i.v. fluid or in the case

**DAILY INTAKE-OUTPUT CHART**

(Not to be filled in Medical Record)

Bodyweight ............................................

24hrs. from ........... on ........... to ........ on .........

| Surname Mr./Mrs./Miss | | Case No. |
|---|---|---|
| First Names | | |

INSTRUCTIONS FOR 24 HOURS (PARENTERAL)
All intravenous fluid therapy and drug additives to these fluids must be prescribed on the "INTRAVENOUS FLUIDS AND DRUG ADDITIVES" form provided. Please refer to this form for fluid volumes which will be required when completing the INTAKE section below. (H.M.R. 111(W) IV).
NOTE The "Type" heading below refers to the particular fluid prescribed in the numbered section on the "INTRAVENOUS FLUID AND DRUG ADDITIVES" form.

INSTRUCTIONS FOR 24 HOURS (ORAL)

| TIME | INTAKE | | | | | | OUTPUT | | | | | |
|---|---|---|---|---|---|---|---|---|---|---|---|---|
| | INTRAVENOUS FLUIDS | | | ORAL | | Other | URINE | | Gastric | | Drainage | Other |
| | Type | Vol. set up | given vol. | Vol. | Type | Vol. | Vol. | S.G. | Vol. | Nature | Vol. | Vol. |
| c/f | | | | | | | | | | | | |
| | | | | | | | | | | | | |
| | | | | | | | | | | | | |
| | | | | | | | | | | | | |
| | | | | | | | | | | | | |
| | | | | | | | | | | | | |
| | | | | | | | | | | | | |
| | | | | | | | | | | | | |
| | | | | | | | | | | | | |
| | | | | | | | | | | | | |
| | | | | | | | | | | | | |
| | | | | | | | | | | | | |
| | | | | | | | | | | | | |
| 24 hour Total | | | | | | | | | | | | |
| | | | | | | | | | | | | |
| | | | | | | | | | | | | |
| | | | | | | | | | | | | |
| | | | | | | | | | | | | |
| | | | | | | | | | | | | |
| | | | | | | | | | | | | |
| | | | | | | | | | | | | |
| | | | | | | | | | | | | |
| | | | | | | | | | | | | |
| | | | | | | | | | | | | |
| | | | | | | | | | | | | |
| | | | | | | | | | | | | |
| 12 hour Total | | | | | | | | | | | | |
| 24 hour Total | | | | | | | | | | | | |

CUMULATIVE BALANCE + − H.M.R. 210A (W)82 (WKJ120X)

**Fig 3.31.1** Fluid balance chart.

of severe illness when capillary membranes become more permeable (leaky). Overload leads to fluid being pushed into interstitial spaces (i.e. spaces outside both cells and vascular system), causing the physical signs of peripheral oedema (may be ankle or whole body oedema) or pulmonary oedema when fluid is pushed into the lungs. Signs and symptoms of pulmonary oedema are shortness of breath, fine crackles on auscultation and 'ground glass' appearance on chest radiograph. If the patient is invasively monitored, there may be changes in CVP, BP and PiCCO® measurements. It is important to distinguish pulmonary oedema from a chest infection as these are managed differently by the physiotherapist.

> *Top tip!*
> What should you consider when trying to distinguish between infection and pulmonary oedema?

## DOCUMENTATION

Urine output and overall fluid balance (Fig. 3.31.1) should be documented under the renal section of your assessment (see Table 2.3, systems-based checklist in Chapter 2) along with a running total of fluid balance. If there are any drains in place (e.g. post-surgery or chest drains) the volume of fluid lost should also be noted. For the unwell patient, it is important to look at a trend over 24 hours rather than the last hour only and consider the pattern over the last few days (e.g. it could be that 4 litres is positive over the last 3 days).

## 3.32 GENERAL OBSERVATION (See CHAPTER 1)

## 3.33 GLASGOW COMA SCALE (GCS)

### DEFINITION

A method for quantifying level of consciousness, it comprises three tests: eye, verbal and motor responses. Although pupil response is not part of this test it is often performed at the same time (see 3.49 Pupils).

### PURPOSE

To monitor changes in neurological function and level of consciousness. It can be used in both the acute and chronic illness settings.

### PROCEDURE

Table 3.33.1 shows how the Glasgow Coma Scale (GCS) is scored. Each element is assessed separately.

- Eyes (E): if the patient is not eye opening spontaneously:
  - ask the patient to open their eyes
  - if the patient does not respond, use a painful stimulus to see if a response can be evoked (see below).

**Table 3.33.1 Glasgow Coma Scale scoring**

| Response | Score |
|---|---|
| **Eye opening** | |
| Opens eyes spontaneously | 4 |
| Opens eyes in response to voice | 3 |
| Opens eyes in response to painful stimuli | 2 |
| Does not open eyes | 1 |
| **Best verbal response** | |
| Orientated, converses normally | 5 |
| Confused, disorientated | 4 |
| Utters inappropriate words | 3 |
| Incomprehensible sounds | 2 |
| Makes no sound | 1 |
| **Best motor response** | |
| Obeys commands | 6 |
| Localizes to painful stimuli | 5 |
| Flexion/withdrawal to painful stimuli | 4 |
| Abnormal flexion to painful stimuli (decorticate) | 3 |
| Extension to painful stimuli (decerebrate) | 2 |
| Makes no movements | 1 |

- Motor (M): note any abnormal patterns of movement shown at rest or on stimulation:
  - ask the patient to stick out their tongue, squeeze your hand or wiggle their toes. Consider the most appropriate option for your patient, e.g. for a patient with a complete spinal injury it would not be appropriate to suggest 'wiggle your toes'.
  - if the patient does not respond, use a painful stimulus to see if a response can be evoked (see below).
- Verbal (V):
  - ask the patient their name
  - note that if the patient is on a ventilator or has a tracheostomy, the score is often 1 in this situation.

Painful stimuli are considered as: a hard object pressed into the nail bed of hands and feet; squeezing the upper trapezius muscles between the thumb and forefinger of the assessor; or supraorbital rub (using the thumb to apply pressure in the top corner of the eye socket). It is no longer recommended to use a sternal rub (rubbing the knuckle of the assessor over the sternum).

### FINDINGS

A normal GCS score is 15/15. The lowest score possible is 3/15. A GCS score of 8 indicates that the patient may be unable to protect their own airway and may require intubation.

When assessing the patient you are looking for best response and any abnormal patterning (e.g. extending or flexing to pain). Deterioration in GCS score should always be highlighted to senior colleagues as this may reflect an acute change in status requiring prompt action.

### DOCUMENTATION

Unless the score is either 3/15 or 15/15, each element of the GCS assessment should be documented, e.g. 'GCS 7/15 (E1, M4, V2)'. Any abnormal patterning should also be noted. This should be recorded in the CNS section of your assessment. Any change in status since the last review or during intervention should be documented.

## 3.34 HEART RATE (HR)

### DEFINITION

Heart rate (HR) is the number of ventricular contractions that occur per minute (beats per minute or b.p.m.). It may be measured by auscultation at the cardiac apex or through an electrocardiograph (ECG). Continuous ECG monitoring may be performed routinely, particularly in critical care (ITU) settings. HR can also be taken manually by palpating one of the body's pulses.

A normal range for HR is 60–100 b.p.m. (at rest).

### PURPOSE

Medically, HR is used as a diagnostic indicator for possible pathologies (e.g. infection or sepsis), to monitor response to treatment and to assess the patient's overall health and fitness (see 3.35 Heart rhythms).

For physiotherapists, HR is measured to assist in deciding whether a patient is stable enough to treat, making decisions regarding exercise tolerance and prescription (see 3.27 Exercise (aerobic fitness) testing), and monitoring response to treatment and possible pain and anxiety. During physiotherapy assessment, it can indicate when to call for help if the patient's HR is abnormal.

## PROCEDURE

Manual pulse can be taken with two fingertips, using light pressure:

- if possible, ensure that the person has been sitting or lying still for at least 5 minutes
- choose an appropriate site.

Some commonly palpated sites are shown in Table 3.34.1. You may count the number of pulsations for 15 seconds and then multiply by 4; however, counting for 60 seconds is recommended for less stable patients in whom HR may be irregular.

Commercial HR monitors are also available, consisting of a chest strap with electrodes. The signal is transmitted to a wrist receiver for display. HR monitors allow accurate measurements to be taken continuously and can be used during exercise when manual measurement would be difficult or impossible (such as when the hands are being used).

## FINDINGS

- *Tachycardia* (>100 b.p.m.): this often occurs with anxiety, exercise (may limit exercise capacity – see 3.27 Exercise (aerobic fitness) testing), fever, anaemia, hypoxia, patients with cardiac disorders and those on certain medications,

**Table 3.34.1 Commonly palpated pulse sites**

| Position | Artery | Reason for use |
| --- | --- | --- |
| Thumb side of wrist | Radial | Easy access pulse and comfortable for individual |
| Medial side of wrist | Ulnar | Not commonly used |
| Neck | Carotid | Strong pulse with easy access |
| Inside of elbow | Brachial | Commonly used with children and babies |
| Groin | Femoral | Use if distal pulse is weak, e.g. hypovolaemia or sepsis |
| Behind medial malleolus | Posterior tibial | Used to check leg perfusion |
| Middle of dorsum of foot | Dorsalis pedis | Used to check leg perfusion |
| Behind the knee | Popliteal | Used to check leg perfusion |
| Over the abdomen | Abdominal aorta | Indicator of abnormal pathology, e.g. abdominal aortic aneurysm |

e.g. bronchodilators and some cardiac drugs may increase HR. A high HR in response to physiotherapy treatment may suggest pain or stress and thus a need to stop or change technique or position.

- *Bradycardia* (<60 b.p.m.): this is seldom symptomatic until below 50 b.p.m. when a person is at total rest. If the patient is feeling well and is not dizzy there is probably no need to be concerned; however, you should report any bradycardia that occurs with symptoms. Also take care when exercising, as HR should normally rise with exercise. Trained athletes tend to have a slow resting HR, and resting bradycardia in athletes should not be considered abnormal if the individual has no symptoms associated with it. Bradycardia may also be caused by some cardiac drugs, especially β-blockers and by vagal nerve stimulation owing to suctioning. If you are unsure whether bradycardia is new or abnormal for the patient, you should seek senior support.

Arrhythmias are abnormalities of the HR and rhythm (sometimes felt by patients as palpitations). They can be divided into two broad categories: fast and slow heart rates. Some cause few or minimal symptoms. Others produce more serious symptoms of light-headedness, dizziness and fainting (see 3.35 Heart rhythms for further information).

In most situations, the HR and pulse rate are identical; a difference between the two is called a 'pulse deficit'. This indicates that some heartbeats have not caused sufficient blood flow to reach the periphery and is commonly found in atrial fibrillation and some other arrhythmias (see 3.35 Heart rhythms).

## DOCUMENTATION

HR should be recorded when documenting a patient's vital signs in the CVS section of the assessment. Any recent changes in HR should also be recorded, especially if there has been a noticeable increase or decrease in the rate. Any changes when undergoing physiotherapy should be documented, as well as the time taken for HR to return to baseline and whether any additional treatment was required to allow the HR to return to baseline.

## 3.35 HEART RHYTHMS

### DEFINITION

Heart rhythm or cardiac rhythm refers to the rhythm of the beating heart and considers the relationship between the atria and ventricles. It is considered alongside heart rate (see 3.34 Heart rate).

## PURPOSE

Assessment of heart rhythms is used to detect many cardiac problems, including angina pectoris, stable angina, ischaemic heart disease, arrhythmias/dysrhythmias (irregular heartbeat), tachycardia (fast heartbeat), bradycardia (slow heartbeat), myocardial infarction (heart attack), and certain congenital heart conditions. Monitoring of heart rhythms is used routinely in physical examinations and for monitoring a patient's condition during and after surgery, as well as in the intensive care setting. Heart rhythm analysis is also used to investigate symptoms such as chest pain, shortness of breath and palpitations (Table 3.35.1 and Figs 3.35.1–3.35.3).

As a physiotherapist you should consider the heart rhythm prior to initiating any treatment. Also the rhythm should be monitored throughout to assess the patient's response to treatment. If any changes in heart rhythm occur then the medical team must be consulted.

## PROCEDURE

Heart rhythms are most commonly measured using an ECG. An ECG is a starting point for detecting many cardiac problems.

An ECG can be completed using either three leads or 12 leads. A three-lead ECG recording is often used within the critical care environment to monitor heart rhythm throughout the course of the day. This provides a guide to heart rhythm but is not as sensitive to change and displays only a small aspect of the heart rhythm. A 12-lead ECG, however, provides a more detailed interpretation of the heart rhythm and is able to detect more discrete changes in myocardial activity.

Both forms of ECG are completed by placing electrodes in specified places on the chest wall (and on the patient's upper and lower limbs for a 12-lead ECG only). The electrodes on different sides of the heart measure the activity of different parts of the heart muscle. The ECG displays the voltage between pairs of these electrodes and hence demonstrates the amount of muscle activity that is occurring. This procedure is rarely completed by physiotherapists.

## FINDINGS

- You are not responsible for diagnosis so always ask for help if unsure!
- Is the patient in a normal sinus rhythm?
- Patients respond differently to dysrhythmias and a serious dysrhythmia in one person may have no adverse effects in another, so look at the patient!
- Blood pressure is the key when deciding the importance of any dysrhythmia (see 3.5 Blood pressure). Also consider general observations such as colour, temperature and level of consciousness.

## Table 3.35.1 Heart rhythms

| Rhythm | Analysis | ECG findings |
|---|---|---|
| Sinus rhythm (SR) | Normal cardiac rhythm proceeding from the sinoatrial node. In healthy adults 60–100 b.p.m. | Consists of a P wave, a QRS complex and a T wave. The P wave is atrial depolarization; the QRS complex occurs as the impulse travels through the ventricles; and the T wave is the repolarization of the ventricles (Fig. 3.35.1) |
| Sinus bradycardia (SB) | See 3.34 Heart rate | A slow rate, regular rhythm, normal QRS complex and the presence of both the P and T wave (Fig. 3.35.1) |
| Sinus tachycardia (ST) | See 3.34 Heart rate | A rapid rate, regular rhythm, normal QRS complex and the presence of both the P and T wave (Fig. 3.35.1) |
| Atrial fibrillation (AF) | Most common arrhythmia, occurring in 5–10% of patients over 65 years. Atrial activity is not sequenced and is mechanically ineffective. The atrioventricular node conducts only a proportion of the atrial impulses to produce irregular ventricular responses. Symptoms range from palpitations and fatigue to acute pulmonary oedema. The area of concern would be fast AF, in which the patient's HR is very high and the blood pressure is compromised | ECG has a rapid rate, irregular heart rhythm and the replacing of P waves with an irregular baseline. (Fig. 3.35.2) |

*(Continued)*

## Table 3.35.1 Heart rhythms—cont'd

| Rhythm | Analysis | ECG findings |
|---|---|---|
| Atrial flutter (A Flutter) | An arrhythmia originating from the atrium. In atrial flutter the atria commonly beat about 300 b.p.m. The atrioventricular node usually conducts every second beat, giving a ventricular rate of 150 b.p.m. Atrial flutter is almost always associated with organic disease of the heart | A mildly irregular baseline trace. Normal QRS complex (Fig. 3.35.2) |
| Atrial ectopic beats (AEB) | Atrial ectopic beats refer to a contraction of the upper heart chamber which occurs before it would be expected. Atrial ectopic beats are also known as premature atrial beats. Patient may not be symptomatic | ECG shows either additional P waves between QRS complexes or an irregular pattern |
| Ventricular tachycardia (VT) | Ventricular tachycardia is defined as three or more consecutive ventricular contractions occurring at a rate of 120 b.p.m. or more. May produce severe hypotension, when urgent DC cardioversion is necessary | ECG shows a rapid ventricular rhythm with broad abnormal QRS complexes (Fig. 3.35.2) |
| Supraventricular tachycardia (SVT) | Any tachycardia that is not ventricular in origin, including normal sinus tachycardia, abnormal sinus tachycardia, ectopic atrial tachycardia, atrial fibrillation/atrial flutter | ECG depends on the cause of SVT (Fig. 3.35.2) |

## 3.35 Heart rhythms

| Rhythm | Analysis | ECG findings |
|---|---|---|
| Ventricular fibrillation (VF) no cardiac output – emergency! | A very rapid and irregular ventricular activation with no mechanical effect and hence no cardiac output. VF rarely reverts spontaneously and requires immediate DC cardioversion | The ECG displays a chaotic wave pattern with no clear T wave, QRS complex or P wave (Fig. 3.35.3) |
| Ventricular ectopic beat (VEB) | An extra heartbeat originating in the lower chamber of the heart. They are common and do not indicate a problem in people without heart disease. However, if a person has aortic stenosis, heart failure, or a previous heart attack, VEBs may be followed by ventricular tachycardia and fibrillation, which can lead to sudden death | ECG shows additional QRS complexes in an irregular pattern |
| Atrioventricular (AV) block (also known as heart block) | Three forms of AV block can be identified – first, second and third degree. The commonest causes are coronary artery disease, cardiomyopathy and fibrosis of the conducting tissue | 1st degree = longer gap between P and R waves<br>2nd degree = QRS does not follow each P wave<br>3rd degree = no coordination between P wave and QRS complex (Fig. 3.35.3) |

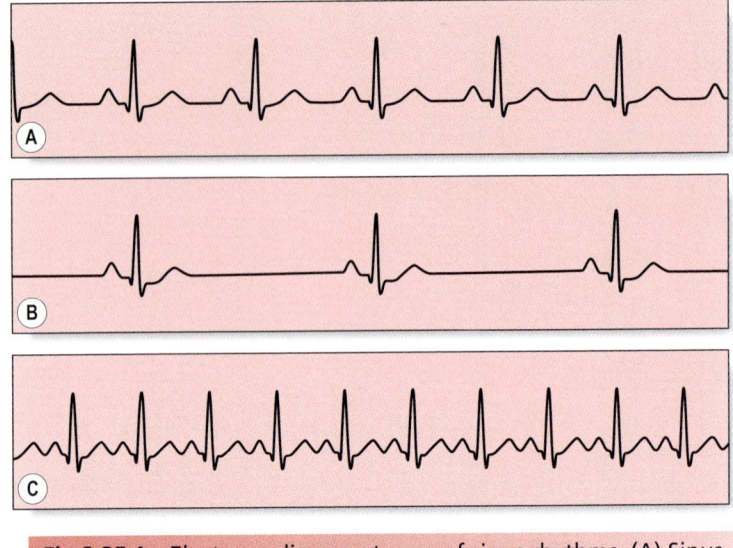

**Fig 3.35.1** Electrocardiogram traces of sinus rhythms. (A) Sinus rhythm. (B) Sinus bradycardia. (C) Sinus tachycardia.

- The trend of any dysrhythmias is also important:
  - Have they just occurred?
  - Did they occur suddenly or gradually?
  - Are the dysrhythmias getting more frequent?
  - How is your treatment affecting them?
  - Pay attention to dysrhythmias that have recently appeared or are getting more frequent.
- Manual chest treatments may affect the ECG tracing, so allow time for the tracing to settle before interpreting any abnormality.
- The most critical heart rhythms are:
  - ventricular tachycardia
  - supraventricular tachycardia
  - ventricular fibrillation – no cardiac output
  - asystole – no cardiac output.

> **Top tip!**
> If you are the first on the scene and the patient has no cardiac output or pulse, activate the buzzer/crash button and start cardiopulmonary resuscitation immediately!

Physiotherapists are not expected to be able to interpret an ECG and are not involved in the management of changes in heart rhythm. However, the presence of heart arrhythmias will have an impact on

## 3.35 Heart rhythms  115

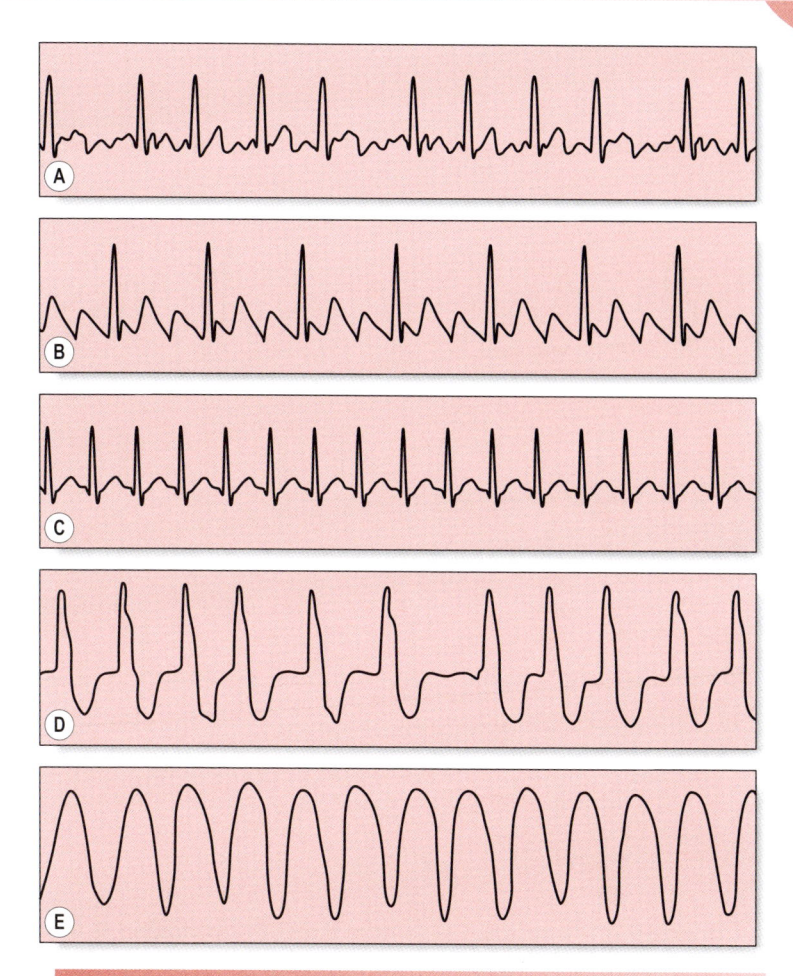

**Fig 3.35.2** Electrocardiogram traces of dysrhythmias. (A) Atrial fibrillation. (B) Atrial flutter. (C) Supraventricular tachycardia. (D,E) Ventricular tachycardia.

whether physiotherapy input is appropriate and whether the patient is able to tolerate treatment. If arrhythmias occur during treatment, medical assistance must be requested and treatment stopped. In some circumstances, the ceasing of treatment may lead to a reversal of the arrhythmias. For further information, see 3.34 Heart rate.

### DOCUMENTATION

When documenting the patient's HR, the rhythm (if known) should also be documented. For example, 'heart rate = 100 b.p.m. (SR)', where SR means sinus rhythm. This then allows for recognition

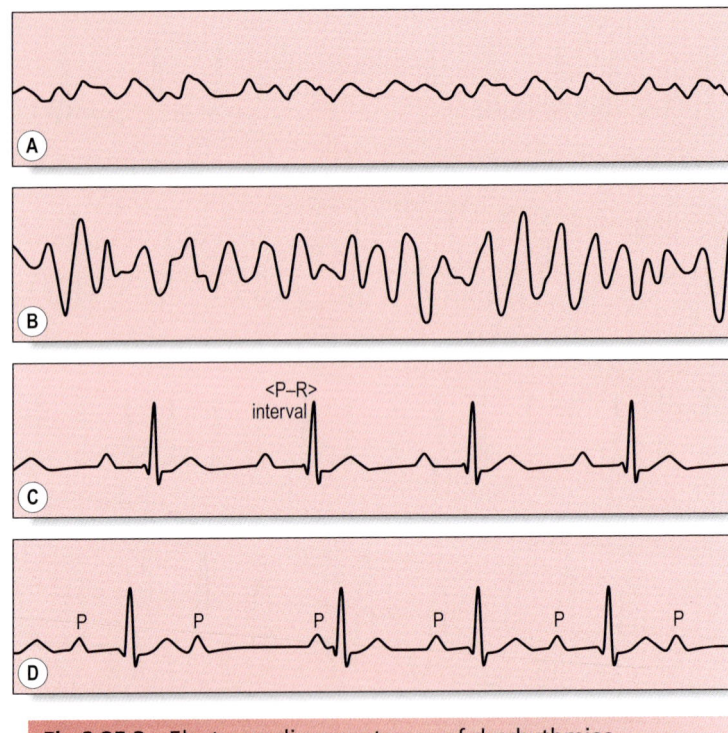

**Fig 3.35.3** Electrocardiogram traces of dysrhythmias. (A,B) Ventricular fibrillation. (C,D) first and second degree heart block.

of deterioration or improvement in a patient's condition as well as considerations for any precautions or contraindications for physiotherapy input. Any changes in HR or rhythm must also be documented and any action taken, e.g. discussion with medical staff.

### 3.36 INSPIRATORY MUSCLE TESTING (See under 3.40 LUNG VOLUMES AND LUNG FUNCTION TESTS – page 120)

### 3.37 INTRACRANIAL PRESSURE (ICP)

#### DEFINITION
The pressure within the cranium that represents the pressure from the brain, blood and cerebrospinal fluid (CSF). It is normally measured in mmHg with a normal resting range of 0–10 mmHg.

## 3.37 Intracranial pressure (ICP)

### PURPOSE

Monitoring ICP allows the team to identify whether the patient's brain is swelling or whether there is pressure being put upon the brain (e.g. following a subarachnoid haemorrhage), which may cause further damage to the brain tissue. It can also monitor whether swelling/pressure is subsiding.

Physiotherapists use ICP as a guide to identify which treatments they can use, as many physiotherapy treatments can have an impact on ICP and CPP, potentially leading to further brain damage (see 3.12 Cerebral perfusion pressure (CPP)).

### PROCEDURE

Medical staff place an ICP probe in the subdural/subarachnoid space under the skull, which gives a continuous digital reading on the monitor by the patient's bedside. ICP may be monitored in one of several ways, as demonstrated in Fig. 3.37.1.

### FINDINGS

The normal value for ICP is 0–10 mmHg; when this value climbs above 20–25 mmHg, the patient may require specialist treatment to reduce ICP.

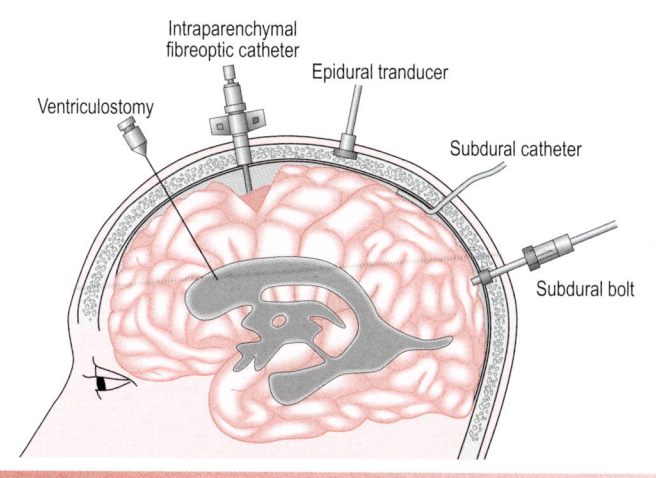

**Fig 3.37.1** Intracranial pressure monitoring.
Reproduced with kind permission from Grant IS, Andrews PJ. 1999 ABC of intensive care: neurological support. British Medical Journal 319: 110–13.

The brain compartment holds three elements – the brain tissue, blood and CSF. If pressure in one element increases, the others must decrease to maintain a stable ICP (Monro–Kellie hypothesis). Following brain injury, ICP may rise.

A raised ICP can be caused by many factors, including neurological deterioration. However, high $P_aCO_2$ and low $P_aO_2$ (perhaps as a result of retained secretions) can also raise ICP as this causes vasodilitation of the blood vessels in the brain; vasodilitation leads to a greater flow of blood to the brain and therefore an increase in ICP. It may be difficult for physiotherapists unfamiliar with this group of patients to decide whether deterioration in the patient's condition is due to neurological or respiratory causes. If you are unsure, it is important that you seek senior advice.

Many physiotherapy treatments can have an impact on ICP and CPP. Increased intrathoracic pressure associated with manual respiratory techniques and manual hyperinflation can reduce venous return to the heart, therefore lowering cardiac output and subsequently BP. A lower BP will lead to a lower MAP, which then affects CPP (see 3.12 Cerebral perfusion pressure (CPP)). Raised intrathoracic pressure may also reduce venous drainage from the head and, therefore, potentially increase ICP. Often the adage 'maximal involvement, minimal intervention' is used, i.e. only treat if treatment is indicated – not just for assessment and not prophylactically.

> *Top tip!*
> Talk with nursing staff about any changes in the patient's ICP in response to nursing procedures, such as turning or washing. If ICP stabilizes quickly after such interventions the patient is likely to tolerate physiotherapy treatment, but if ICP takes 2–3 hours to stabilize, physiotherapy might not be tolerated well. Seek senior advice prior to treating potentially unstable patients.

### DOCUMENTATION

The ICP value should be documented under the CNS section of assessment and should be considered alongside the global clinical picture. Any changes in ICP during treatment must be recorded along with the time it took to return to baseline and whether any action was required by nursing or medical staff to rectify the change.

## 3.38 ITU (CRITICAL CARE) CHARTS

### DEFINITION
The 24 hour spreadsheet on which ITU nurses document hourly key observations within the critical care setting.

### PURPOSE
Charts within critical care vary between institutions; however, there is a general overview that is common to many. Fig. 3.38.1 may help you locate the information you are seeking to aid your assessment.

### PROCEDURE
ITU nurses document observations on the chart over a period of time – usually over a 24 hour period – and these observations are usually recorded every hour. The value of these charts is that you can see what has happened to the patient over a period of time. This facilitates spotting trends and also linking changes in one system to changes in another, e.g. if RR increases, has there been any change in HR?

It should be noted that documentation using ITU-type charts is common practice within high-care/dependency areas and the format of charting may be very similar to this.

### DOCUMENTATION
What should be documented within a critical care assessment can be seen in Chapter 2, Table 2.5 Critical care/ITU patients.

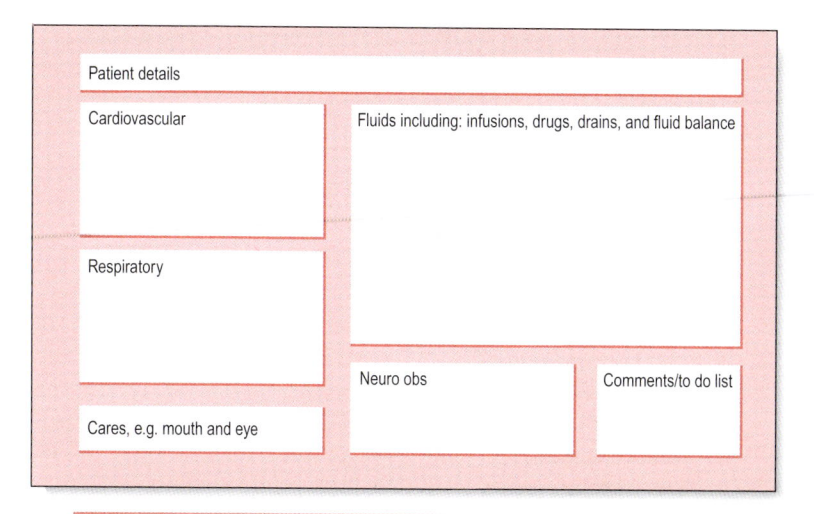

| Patient details | |
|---|---|
| Cardiovascular | Fluids including: infusions, drugs, drains, and fluid balance |
| Respiratory | |
| | Neuro obs / Comments/to do list |
| Cares, e.g. mouth and eye | |

**Fig 3.38.1** Example of an ITU/critical care chart.

## 3.39 LEVEL OF CONSCIOUSNESS (SEE ALSO 3.4 AVPU, 3.33 GLASGOW COMA SCALE AND 3.57 SEDATION/AGITATION SCORE)

### DEFINITION
A measure of how responsive a patient is to the environment, stimuli or the degree of arousal.

### PURPOSE
To ascertain the patient's ability to participate in treatment. It can also be used as a marker of progression or deterioration (for further information, see 3.4 AVPU, 3.33 Glasgow Coma Scale and 3.57 Sedation/agitation score).

### PROCEDURE
Observe the patient and attempt to rouse them by asking them to respond to simple questioning; consider the appropriateness of their response.

> **Top tip!**
> If a patient has a less than normal conscious level, find out whether this is recent. Any sudden or recent deterioration should be reported and may need urgent intervention.

### DOCUMENTATION
In the absence of using AVPU, GCS or a sedation score it is acceptable to note the patient's level of awareness; this should be done in the CNS section of your assessment, e.g. awake and alert/very sleepy/appears confused.

## 3.40 LUNG VOLUMES AND LUNG FUNCTION TESTS (PULMONARY FUNCTION TESTS)

### DEFINITION
The measurement of ventilation (movement of air into and out of the lungs) during normal and/or maximal breathing manoeuvres.

Volumes and/or flow rates of inspired or expired air may be measured by portable equipment in GPs' surgeries, hospital wards and clinics (spirometry) and even in the patient's own home. However, measurements of the volumes (static volumes), volumes between breaths and other tests such as muscle function pressures and gas transfer can only be made by specialized equipment in the

## 3.40 Lung volumes and lung function tests

pulmonary function laboratory. The most commonly measured test that physiotherapists may need to be able to either conduct or interpret is spirometry in order to find the forced vital capacity (FVC), forced expiratory volume in the first second ($FEV_1$) and peak expiratory flow rate (PEFR). These are dynamic volumes. Definitions of all these volumes and measurements are described in Tables 3.40.1 and 3.40.2 and discussed under Findings.

Inspiratory muscle testing can be performed; however, testing is dependent on the effort of the patient and, therefore, the level of reliability or reproducibility may not be consistent. As this measurement is less commonly used in practice, results have not been discussed under Findings.

### PURPOSE

There are a number of reasons to review lung volumes and lung function tests (LFTs):

- to look for the presence of lung disease and aid diagnosis
- to grade the severity of respiratory disorders
- to differentiate between different pathologies

**Table 3.40.1 Key terms in normal respiratory mechanics**

| | Lung volumes |
|---|---|
| Tidal volume | The volume of a normal resting breath |
| Inspiratory reserve volume | The extra volume that can be inhaled after a normal inspiratory breath to reach maximal inspiration |
| Expiratory reserve volume | The extra volume that can be exhaled after a normal expiratory breath to reach maximal expiration |
| Residual volume | The amount of air left in the lungs after full expiration – this cannot be directly measured |
| Vital capacity | The volume from maximal inspiration to maximal expiration |
| Functional residual capacity | The amount of air left in the lungs at the end of a normal tidal volume – this cannot be directly measured |
| Total lung capacity | The total volume of the lung if completely emptied and includes the residual volume – this cannot be directly measured |

**Table 3.40.2 Dynamic lung function tests measure volumes over a period of time**

| | |
|---|---|
| PEFR or PEF | Peak expiratory flow rate or peak expiratory flow is the highest flow rate achieved with forced expiration following a maximal inspiration. It can be measured with very small, cheap and simple flow meters which may be given to patients to use at home. It is often used as an indicator of airflow obstruction in asthma |
| $FEV_1$ | The volume of air a subject can exhale in the first second of a maximal breath out, following a maximal inspiration |
| Forced vital capacity (FVC) | The volume expired forcefully (following a maximal inspiration), until residual volume is reached |
| $FEV_1$/FVC | Looks at the amount of air expelled within the first second compared with the overall volume achieved |
| Flow–volume loop/curve | This procedure starts from tidal breath in, then measures a full inspiration followed immediately by a forced maximal expiration. The curve is plotted from rates at specific volumes |

- to monitor disease progression over time
- to evaluate the response to treatment (e.g. response to bronchodilators or steroids).

Physiotherapists may occasionally be required to take these measurements and may also need to interpret LFT results in order to determine disease progression. It may also be useful for physiotherapists to distinguish between restrictive and obstructive lung disease (this is discussed further under Findings) in order to select appropriate treatments. For example, patients with low lung volumes may require deep breathing exercises or positions to increase ventilation.

### *PROCEDURE*
- *PEFR*: the patient is asked to take a maximal breath in and then blow out forcefully into a peak flow meter. This is a short and sharp manoeuvre. The figure recorded is normally the best of three attempts.
- *Spirometry*: the patient is asked to take a maximal breath in and then blow out forcefully into a device and keep blowing until they can exhale no more. They will be asked to repeat this to ensure a consistent result. This test measures $FEV_1$ and FVC.

See the guidelines in Further reading for more detailed instructions on performing these tests, including safety measures.

## 3.40 Lung volumes and lung function tests

### FINDINGS

The primary function of the lung is gas exchange. This is achieved using three physiological mechanisms:

- *Ventilation*: the bulk movement of gas in and out of the lungs.
- *Diffusion*: the movement of a substance from an area of high concentration to an area of low concentration along a gradient.
- *Perfusion*: the movement of blood through the pulmonary circulation.

Breathing moves gas in and out of the lungs; the thin membrane of the lung and large surface area facilitate diffusion, and the constant supply of blood transports oxygen from the lungs to the body and returns carbon dioxide for removal.

There are a variety of methods to measure the efficiency of these mechanisms and compare them with normal values in a laboratory setting; however, there will be a focus on simple bedside tests in this section. Lung function tests focus on the ventilation component only; for more detail on background respiratory physiology and testing, the reader is directed to the Further reading.

Table 3.40.1 and Fig. 3.40.1 set out the static volumes that can be measured in the physiology laboratory. It is important to understand these first before going on to look at the dynamic values that are commonly measured in the clinics and hospital wards (Table 3.40.2).

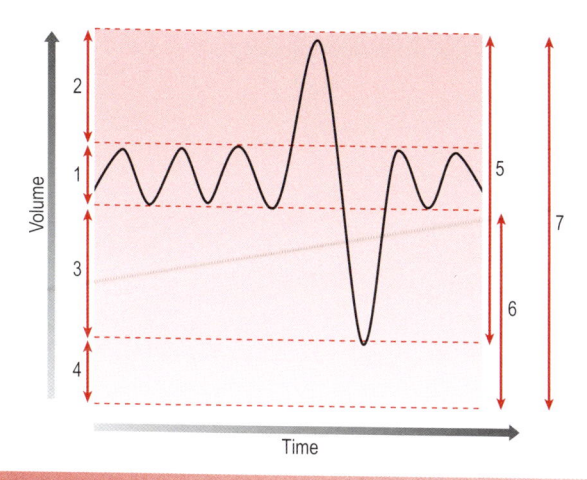

**Fig 3.40.1** Static lung volumes. 1 = Tidal Volume; 2 = Inspiratory Reserve Volume; 3 = Expiratory Reserve Volume; 4 = Residual Volume; 5 = Vital Capacity; 6 = Functional Residual Capacity; 7 = Total Lung Capacity

The results are compared with the predicted result for a patient of the same age, sex, height and ethnic origin and the result is converted into a percentage; for example,

(measured FVC = 4.5 / predicted FVC = 6.0) × 100 = 75%

Any result below 80% or above 120% of predicted is considered to be outside the normal range. Below 80% of predicted is suggestive of pathology. If previous values are available, they provide a useful comparison to review disease progression.

### How to interpret abnormal lung function testing
- Is the FVC normal? If the FVC is lower than 80% predicted this suggests pathology; however, at this point it is not possible to decide whether this is an obstructive or a restrictive problem.
- Is $FEV_1$ normal? If the $FEV_1$ is less than 80% of predicted this also suggests pathology. However, if considered on its own it is not possible to say whether this is a restrictive or obstructive problem.
- Is the $FEV_1/FVC$ ratio normal?

### Identify an obstructive problem
- Airflow obstruction: there is a partial block or narrowing of the conducting airways and the patient is having difficulty getting air out of the lung quickly. This results in a flattened spirogram (Fig. 3.40.2). Look at the $FEV_1/FVC \times 100$ ratio. Any value lower than 70% suggests obstructive respiratory disease such as asthma or COPD.

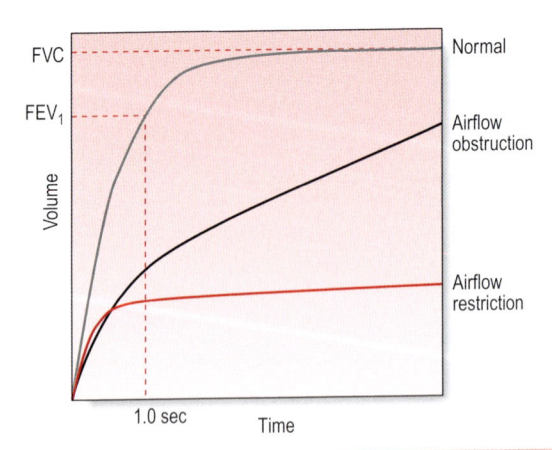

**Fig 3.40.2** A simplified graph to demonstrate a spirogram, with forced vital capacity in first second of expiration ($FEV_1$) and forced vital capacity (FVC) demonstrated.

### Identify a restrictive problem
- Airflow restriction (Fig. 3.40.2): here the total volume of air the patient is able to blow out is limited (so the FVC would be low), but there is no obstruction (so the $FEV_1/FVC$ ratio is above 70%). This happens because the patient is not able to take in a deep enough breathe initially, which then reduces the FVC. The air that they do manage to expire will come out quickly, so the $FEV_1/FVC$ ratio can be high. This would be found in patients with kyphoscoliosis – a non-reversible condition – or a pleural effusion which could be drained.

### Combined problems
- Some patients have both a reduced FVC AND $FEV_1$ together with a lower $FEV_1/FVC$ ratio – they may be classified as having obstructive AND restrictive problems.
- Flow volume loop: inspiratory curves can indicate muscle strength and vocal cord problems. Expiratory loops are good indicators for extrathoracic obstruction and small airway blockage.

## DOCUMENTATION

The results for $FEV_1$ and FVC are expressed in litres and PEFR is expressed in litres per minute. The $FEV_1/FVC$ ratio is always expressed as a percentage. These should be documented under the respiratory heading of your assessment.

## FURTHER READING

American Association for Respiratory Care, 1996. AARC Clinical Practice Guideline Spirometry, 1996 Update. Respir. Care 41, 629–36.

Cotes, J.E., 1993. Lung Function Assessment and Application to Medicine. Blackwell Scientific Publications, Oxford, UK (Chapter 6).

Quanjer, P.H., Tammeling, G.J., Cotes, J.E., et al, 1993. Lung volumes and forced ventilatory flows. Eur. Respir. J. 6 (Suppl. 16), 5–40.

West, J.B., 2008. Respiratory Physiology: The Essentials, 8th edn. Lippincott, Williams and Wilkins, Baltimore, MD.

## 3.41 MUSCLE CHARTING (OXFORD GRADING)

### DEFINITION

A form of manual muscle testing which assesses the power of a muscle. This is then rated on a scale (0–5) to provide an objective marker.

## PURPOSE

It is important for a physiotherapist to measure muscle strength as objectively as possible when assessing an individual. This is completed to obtain a baseline level from which future improvement or deterioration can be measured. This allows the therapist to devise an individual exercise plan and to evaluate its effectiveness.

The Oxford scale provides an indication of the strength of a particular muscle or group of muscles. It is relatively quick and easy to complete and requires no equipment, and as such it is widely used in all areas of clinical practice.

However, the scale is limited as it is subjective, and is not functional or sensitive to change since the movements resisted are concentric contractions. Also, the spaces between the grades are not linear (Table 3.41.1).

## PROCEDURE

For information on muscle strength testing for particular joints and/or muscles refer to Fox and Day (2009) (see Further reading).

## FINDINGS

- Grade 0: no action discernible in the muscle belly or tendon when the patient attempts to perform the activity several times.
- Grade 1: twitch discerned as the muscle undergoes a small contraction but is not strong enough to perform any of its specified joint movement.
- Grade 2: muscle is strong enough to perform its designated joint movement when the force of gravity is eliminated (making it much easier to perform). The joint must be accurately positioned for this to be tested correctly.
- Grade 3: muscle is strong enough to perform the joint action to the full range against gravity but with no resistance applied. An example is a patient lifting his or her arm above their head.

Table 3.41.1 Oxford grading scale

| Grade | Definition |
|---|---|
| 0 | No contraction of the muscle |
| 1 | A flicker of a contraction |
| 2 | Full range of movement with gravity eliminated |
| 3 | Full range of movement against gravity and with a hold |
| 4 | Full range of movement against a minimal resistance |
| 5 | Full range of movement against a maximal resistance |

- Grade 4: muscle can move the joint through the full movement both against gravity and against some resistance such as body weight or gentle resistance applied by the therapist. It is a professional judgment as to the resistance to be applied for the test, and the physiotherapist should have in mind the health, age, activity and weight of the patient.
- Grade 5: the patient's normal power, but as this will vary greatly between individuals the physiotherapist must make an estimation of the expected full muscle power for that particular patient. Grade 5 for a frail sick person will be very different from grade 5 for a young, fit, sports person.

To demonstrate the subjectivity of this measurement some therapists may also use a '+' or '−' after the grade. If the patient can raise their arm up above the head to some extent but not very strongly nor to full range, the physiotherapist might grade that as 3/5 for the deltoid muscle but, because it is not full, it might be rated 3−/5. If the muscle will take good manual resistance but does not appear to be normal for that patient then the grading could be 4+/5.

This grading scale allows the physiotherapist to test all the appropriate muscles and record them in the patient's notes, enabling progress to be charted against time as the strength improves.

### DOCUMENTATION

When documenting Oxford grading it is essential to record the muscle being tested, the patient's starting position (e.g. long sitting) and the estimated muscle power from 0/5 to 5/5. This information is required to ensure that the test can reliably be repeated for that given patient and that given muscle group.

Any observations made during the test should also be recorded, e.g. any noticeable loss of range, pain or abnormal movement pattern.

### FURTHER READING

Fox, J., Day, R., 2009. A Physiotherapist's Guide to Clinical Measurement. Churchill Livingstone, Edinburgh, UK.

## 3.42 MYOTOMES (SEE ALSO 3.41 MUSCLE CHARTING (OXFORD GRADING))

### DEFINITION

A myotome is a muscle that is supplied by one main spinal nerve root (Fig. 3.42.1). It is the motor equivalent of a dermatome. Myotome assessment can be used to assess peripheral nerve injuries and spinal cord injuries.

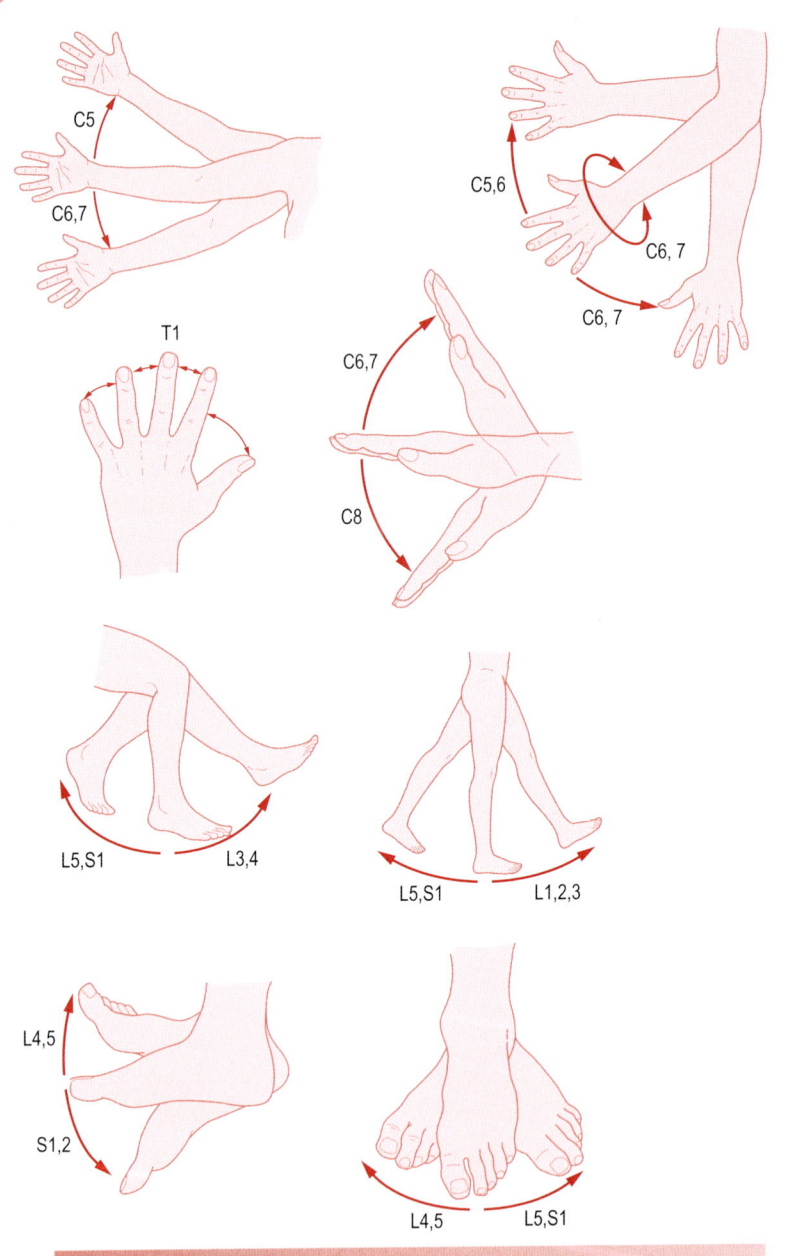

**Fig 3.42.1** Myotomes.
Reproduced with kind permission from Crossman AR, Neary D. 2002 Neuroanatomy: An Illustrated Colour Text, 2nd Edn. Edinburgh, UK: Churchill Livingstone.

## PURPOSE

Myotome testing is designed to test the integrity of the nerve supply to a group of muscles. A muscle group's isometric muscle strength relates directly to the nerve root innervations, and thus may aid in the identification of the potential nerve root lesion.

## PROCEDURE

The procedure is fully described in Day et al (2009) (see Further reading).

## FINDINGS

Weakness or inability to contract individual muscles provides a guide to the level of injury. In practice, within the cardiorespiratory setting, it should be noted that 'C3, 4 and 5 keep the diaphragm alive' and that abdominal muscles are highly important for an effective cough. Thus, any injury above and including the thoracic level can have an impact on respiratory function.

As with dermatomes, it may be necessary to re-chart myotomes on several occasions to assess improvement or deterioration in level of function. This is particularly relevant in the management of early spinal injury in which 'spinal shock' (i.e. inflammatory response in the spinal cord) may cause a higher level of deficit than the original injury level. This needs to be closely monitored.

## DOCUMENTATION

See 3.41 Muscle charting (Oxford grading) for documentation.

## FURTHER READING

Day, R., Fox, J., Paul-Taylor, G., 2009. Neuro-musculoskeletal Clinical Testing: A Clinician's Guide. Churchill Livingstone, Edinburgh, UK.

## 3.43 OXYGEN DELIVERY

### DEFINITION

Oxygen therapy is the administration of oxygen at concentrations greater than that in ambient air (i.e. above 21%) to treat or prevent the symptoms and problems associated with hypoxia. It is used to achieve normal or near-normal tissue oxygenation, without causing a reduction in ventilation and consequent increase in arterial carbon dioxide tension or oxygen toxicity.

Oxygen therapy can be provided in both the acute and community environment to assist in the management of hypoxaemia.

## PURPOSE

Oxygen is a drug and should be prescribed by a medical professional; however, physiotherapists need to assess oxygen delivery to ensure that the patient is receiving the amount of oxygen that has been prescribed. The physiotherapist may also assess whether oxygen therapy is sufficient and whether the modality by which it is delivered is appropriate. They need to monitor oxygen delivery during exercise or physiotherapy treatment and may (depending on the setting) be allowed to alter oxygen delivery in response to changes in oxygen saturation.

## PROCEDURE

Oxygen can be delivered to a patient in several different ways (Fig. 3.43.1). Physiotherapists are not normally involved in the prescription of oxygen but in an emergency situation are allowed to increase oxygen as needed and change the method of delivery. The most common methods of delivery are:

- nasal cannulae or specs
- face mask – simple or Venturi or non-rebreathe mask
- tracheostomy mask
- ventilator
- resuscitation bag
- head box (small children).

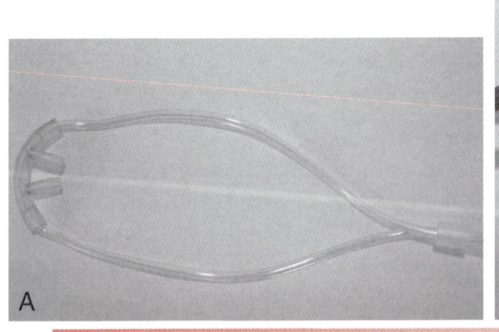

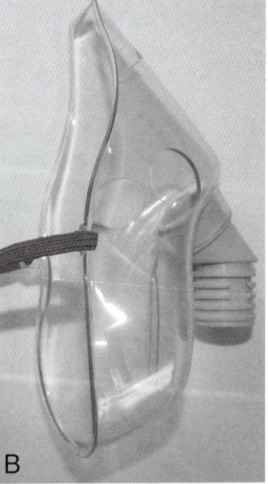

**Fig 3.43.1** Oxygen delivery devices. A, nasal cannula; B, simple face mask;

## 3.43 Oxygen delivery

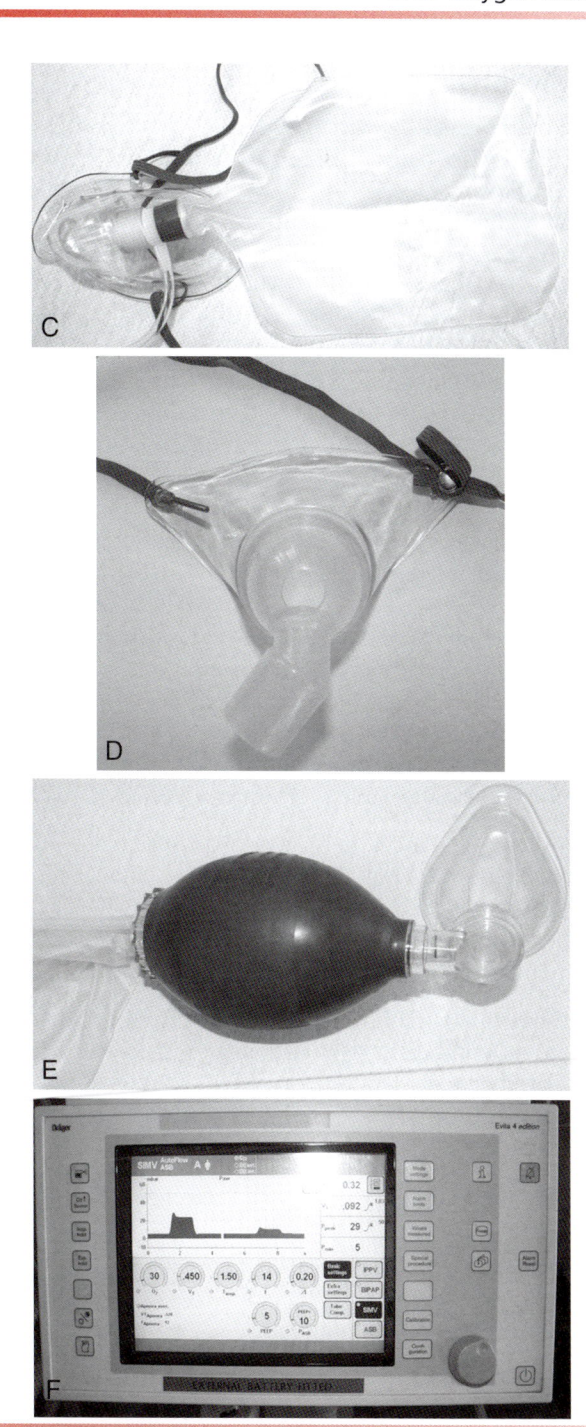

**Fig 3.43.1, cont'd** C, non-rebreathe mask; D, tracheostomy mask; E, Ambu bag; F, ventilator.

Oxygen delivery is divided into two main categories:

- Fixed performance devices (high flow):
  - These masks deliver oxygen at a rate above the peak inspiratory flow rate.
  - They deliver fixed concentrations of oxygen, e.g. Venturi face mask, and are necessary particularly for patients with reduced hypoxic drives (e.g. COPD patients) and those with type II respiratory failure (see 3.1 Arterial blood gases).
  - They deliver an accurate percentage of oxygen (24–60%).
  - Correct oxygen flow is important.
  - Table 3.43.1 summarizes the flow required for each percentage oxygen – the % and flow rate required is also marked on individual valves.
- Variable flow devices (low and variable flow):
  - These devices deliver oxygen at less than the peak inspiratory flow rate and therefore provide a variable concentration of oxygen.
  - The percentage of oxygen delivered is dependent on the rate and depth of the patient's respiration.
  - Suitable for patients who do not require an accurate percentage of oxygen.
  - Table 3.43.2 summarizes flow rates and the potential concentrations of variable performance devices.

In many circumstances it may be appropriate to add humidification to the oxygen delivery system. This may help sputum clearance, as it will prevent the drying effects of oxygen. Humidification can be added using any of the following equipment:

- heat moisture exchanger: used for ventilated patients
- heated humidification systems, e.g. Fisher Paykell: used for ventilated patients

Table 3.43.1 Venturi valves

| Venturi valve | Oxygen flow |
| --- | --- |
| 24% (blue) | 2 l/min |
| 28% (white) | 4 l/min |
| 35% (yellow) | 8 l/min |
| 40% (red) | 10 l/min |
| 60% (green) | 15 l/min |

## 3.43 Oxygen delivery

Table 3.43.2 Variable flow devices

| Delivery system | Concentration | Flow rate | Additional information |
| --- | --- | --- | --- |
| Non-rebreathe mask | 60–90% (dependent on breathing pattern) | 15 l/min | Can be very dry – causing dry secretions |
| Simple face mask | 40–60% | 1–15 l/min | Flow rates <5 l/min can lead to $CO_2$ retention |
| Nasal cannula | Low–medium dose | 1–4 l/min | Patients likely to experience nasal dryness with higher flow rate |

- cold water large volume nebulizers, e.g. Hudson or Respi-flo
- cold water bubble-through systems
- saline nebulizers.

### FINDINGS

The concentration of oxygen being delivered to the patient is a key indicator of the clinical condition. Patients on higher oxygen requirements normally have a worse clinical picture. Also, patients who have had sudden increases in oxygen demand are likely to be deteriorating and require referral to the medical team. The patient may require either a change in concentration of oxygen or a change in delivery system (e.g. change from nasal cannula to face mask if the patient is mostly mouth breathing).

Changes in oxygen therapy can also assist in the decision as to whether physiotherapy input is required and how likely the patient is to tolerate the intervention. You should be aware of a patient's oxygen requirements prior to initiating any form of intervention and, if appropriate, monitor oxygen saturations during the treatment. Physiotherapists will also be involved in suggesting the use of humidification with oxygen therapy (e.g. patients with viscous secretions).

### DOCUMENTATION

Level of oxygen and method of delivery should be noted in the respiratory section of your assessment. In the community setting, the duration that the oxygen therapy is in use should also be documented. These patients can be using long-term oxygen therapy for up to 24 hours each day.

## ASSESSMENT TOOLS

It must also be documented whether additional oxygen therapy was provided during a physiotherapy assessment or treatment session and also whether the oxygen delivery device was altered or changed as part of the physiotherapy session.

## 3.44 PAIN SCORE

### DEFINITION

Pain is subjective and as healthcare professionals we should accept that pain is what the patient tells us. Pain scores quantify the patient's perspective of pain severity and may be done by verbal report, through pointing to scales or pictures or (if a patient is unable to express themselves) based on the behaviour of the patient.

An example of a pain scoring chart is shown in Table 3.44.1.

### PURPOSE

Pain scores are used to evaluate the patient's response to pain-relieving medication and to identify deterioration or improvement. If pain is not well controlled, this can lead to postoperative complications similar to those associated with immobility and respiratory compromise.

### PROCEDURE

Ask the patient to rate their level of pain severity out of 3 (where 0 = no pain and 3 is the worst pain they could imagine). Some units use a scale of 0–10.

Patients with speech problems and children may be asked to point to a picture (or scale) that represents their pain.

If the patient is unable to indicate their pain severity (e.g. because they are unconscious), the assessor may estimate pain relief based on behaviour.

**Table 3.44.1 Pain scoring chart**

| Ask the patient 'Which word describes best the pain you have when you move?' | |
|---|---|
| No pain | 0 |
| Mild pain | 1 |
| Moderate pain | 2 |
| Severe pain | 3 |

### FINDINGS
Be aware of physiological responses to pain, which include increased HR, BP and RR. Therefore, if these parameters are deranged, it is important to consider the option that pain relief may not be effective during our assessment.

Note any deterioration and determine whether pain levels are acceptable. If pain is not well controlled, patients will not be able to participate in assessment or treatment and this may lead to complications.

### DOCUMENTATION
Note the route of analgesia (e.g. epidural, patient-controlled analgesia) and if pain control is adequate.

## 3.45 PALPATION

### DEFINITION
Palpation involves using your hands to assess the patient's breathing pattern, abdomen and limbs.

### PURPOSE
- To supplement observations of breathing pattern, and help to identify:
  - degree of expansion
  - work of breathing
  - sputum retention
  - pain or tenderness
  - changes in temperature
  - any swelling (oedema) in the area.
- To communicate with the patient and gain their confidence.
- To identify any circulatory problems, hypothermia or fever.

### PROCEDURE (Fig. 3.45.1)
Place your hands comfortably on each of these areas in turn:

- neck and shoulder girdle
- apical (over upper ribs and upper chest area)
- lateral costal (over lower ribs and lower chest area)
- abdominal (diaphragmatic).

Palpate each area during resting breathing and repeat for deep (full) inspiration:

- use your hands to feel for depth of movement and equality of expansion during resting and maximal breathing
- note the quality and smoothness of movement and coordination between the chest and abdomen

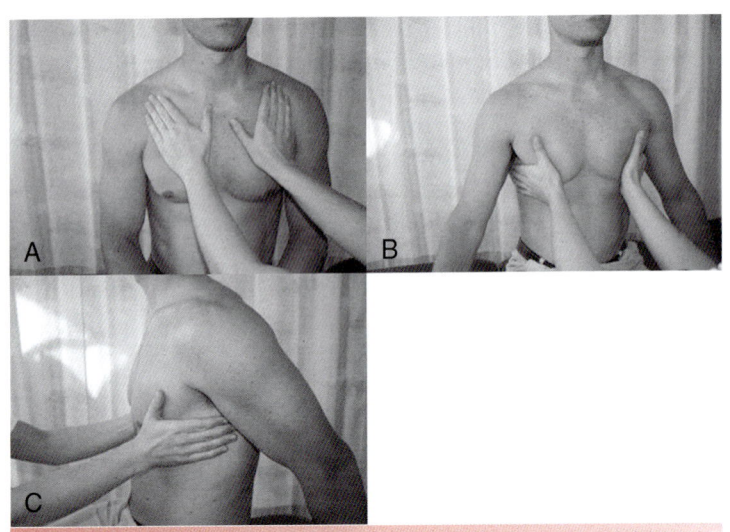

**Fig 3.45.1** Chest wall palpation. (A) Apical palpation. (B) Basal palpation (front view). (C) Basal palpation (side view).

- note any pain, increased muscle tension, tenderness or swelling, or sputum movement in the area
- feel the hands and feet for altered temperature and/or swelling.

### FINDINGS
Consider auscultation findings as well when interpreting what you feel.

### Thorax and respiratory movement
- Palpation may be used to support your observations of RR and breathing pattern.
- Presence of secretions may be felt as crackles over the affected lung fields during breathing, particularly during expiration. Beware of very shallow breathers – these crackles may not be as obvious. Asking patients to breathe out through their mouth and to breathe more deeply may sometimes help to determine whether secretions are present as they may be more easily heard.

> **Top tip!**
> If you feel secretions, you may need to address these straight away. If they are significantly obstructing the airway you should clear them before continuing with the rest of your assessment.

- Pain or tenderness may indicate recent injury or infection – manual techniques may need caution or may be contraindicated.

- Note any sign of surgical emphysema (a popping feeling like bubble wrap directly under the skin); this might be related to internal damage or pneumothorax and should be reported. Manual techniques may need caution or be contraindicated and positive pressure should be avoided.
- Paradoxical movements – inward movements of the lower ribs during inspiration may be due to ineffective diaphragmatic contraction secondary to hyperinflation in patients with COPD. Poor coordination between abdominal movements and rib cage movements may suggest diaphragmatic fatigue, and the possibility of impending respiratory failure.

## Abdomen
- If the abdomen is tight, tense or tender it may be inhibiting the movement of the diaphragm and restricting breathing.
- In the surgical patient an 'open abdomen' may occur, where the incision site is not closed. Noting this is important as this will affect the patient's ability to cough and he/she may not be appropriate to mobilize.

## Upper and lower limb
- Cold peripheries (especially if they feel clammy) may be due to significant circulatory disorders that require immediate intervention (e.g. circulatory shock).
- Dryness in the axilla may be due to dehydration, particularly if accompanied by a dry mouth and a drop in urine output.
- Bilateral lower limb oedema may be related to right-sided heart failure or overhydration.
- Warm skin may be due to $CO_2$ retention (hypercapnia). Warm, sweaty feel may indicate infection or anxiety.

### DOCUMENTATION
Describe what you have felt, specifying whether left or right sided.

### 3.46 PEAK FLOW (See under 3.40 LUNG VOLUMES AND LUNG FUNCTION TESTS – page 120)

### 3.47 PERCUSSION NOTE

### DEFINITION
The sound heard when striking the chest wall briskly with the fingers to detect the presence or absence of air in the thorax.

## PURPOSE

This technique is particularly useful (along with other clinical findings) for indicating pleural effusion, consolidation, emphysema or pneumothorax.

## PROCEDURE

- Place the fingers of your non-dominant hand flat along the chest wall in between the ribs, with slightly hyperextended fingers and a firm pressure. Strike the middle finger with the middle fingertip of your cupped dominant hand with a 'bouncing' action caused by a flick of the wrist. (This technique is the same as when 'sounding' a wall to see if it is hollow (plasterboard) or solid; Fig. 3.47.1.)
- Repeat the process in a systematic manner over the lung fields as with auscultation (see 3.3 Auscultation) and note the degree of resonance you feel/hear.

### Top tip!

Practise your percussion technique over normal lung tissue (resonant), then compare this by percussing over the liver or the clavicle (dull). This will help you to differentiate between the two sounds.

## FINDINGS

- A dull sound and a solid feel (like tapping on a brick wall) suggests absence of air in the region, e.g. when percussing over the liver (right anterior, subcostal).

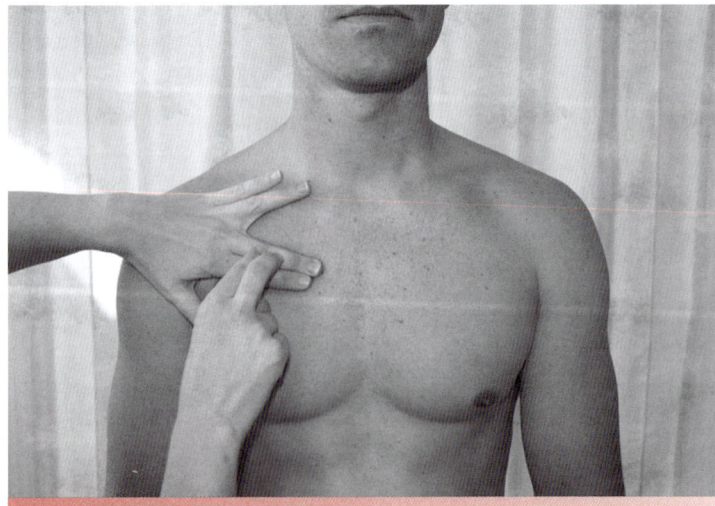

**Fig 3.47.1** Percussion technique.

- A resonant sound and a vibrant feel (like tapping on a stud/plasterboard wall) suggests the presence of air in the region, e.g. when percussing over the lung fields.
- If you percuss over lung tissue but the sound and feel is more like over the liver, this suggests absence of air in that region, which could be due to consolidation (as with lobar pneumonia), lung collapse or pleural effusion.
- If your percussion sounds very resonant (more so than usual, or more than the same lung zone on the opposite side), this is called 'hyper-resonant' (or 'tympanic' as it has a slightly musical quality) and suggests more air in the lung or pleural space. This could be due to hyperinflation as in emphysema or asthma or, if only on one side, a pneumothorax.
- Consider alongside auscultation findings.

### DOCUMENTATION

Record the resonance (e.g. dull, resonant or hyper-resonant) in different lung zones (e.g. anterior or posterior, upper, middle or lower lobes).

## 3.48 PULSE OXIMETRY

### DEFINITION

Pulse oximetry is the non-invasive measurement of estimated saturation of arterial Hb with oxygen. The pulse oximeter has a probe that can be attached to the fingertip or ear lobe that senses and displays the patient's pulse rate (HR) and oxygen saturations. Light generated by the probe is absorbed by Hb in the pulsating capillary (approximating arterial blood) in a pattern that depends on its percentage saturation with oxygen. This is calculated and displayed as the $S_pO_2$ (oxygen saturation of pulsating blood), also known as saturations (or sats) (Fig. 3.48.1). Saturations (sats) can also be measured directly (invasively) from arterial blood and recorded as $S_aO_2$ (see 3.1 Arterial blood gases).

### PURPOSE

Oximetry allows for continuous monitoring of $S_pO_2$ in the critically ill patient. It can be used to monitor the patient's response to exercise and activity in hospital and community settings. It can also be used to make treatment decisions (e.g. the need for oxygen therapy; see 3.43 Oxygen delivery), ensuring safety/effectiveness of interventions (e.g. position change), as an outcome measure (e.g. following manual chest clearance) and to aid exercise prescription.

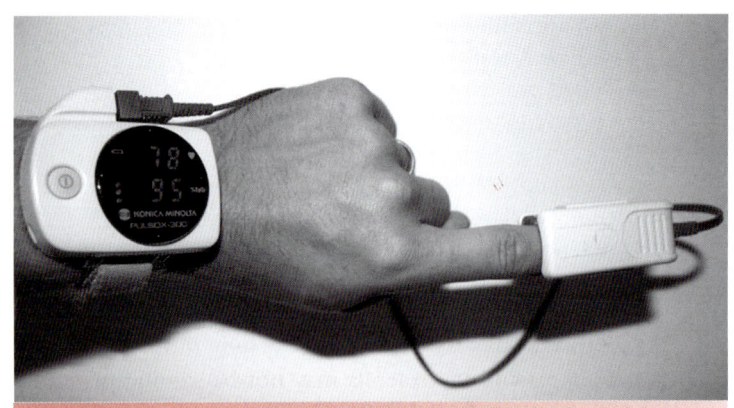

**Fig 3.48.1** A portable pulse oximeter with finger probe. Note on the display read out, the top figure is heart rate and the bottom figure is $S_pO_2$.

## PROCEDURE
- Clean the probe with appropriate wipes.
- Check that the patient's finger is clean and remove any dark nail polish.
- Ask the patient to rest his/her hand (e.g. on their upper abdomen or chest) and remain still to prevent movement 'artefacts' affecting the measurement.
- Check that the finger is pink and warm – rub the finger to warm it if necessary.
- Place the probe over the fingertip with the light emission point next to the fingernail.
- Check that the probe is picking up the HR accurately compared with the manual pulse.

It can sometimes take some time for the machine to settle and get an accurate reading. In the acute setting, if the reading is not normal for the patient, you should seek help as the patient may be acutely unwell and need prompt attention.

If leaving the patient unattended with the device, check that the alarms are set appropriately.

## FINDINGS
$S_pO_2$ tells you how 'full' the Hb is but does not necessarily tell you whether a patient does or does not have enough oxygen, because this will also depend on the amount of functioning Hb present. Patients with anaemia have less Hb, so, even with a $S_pO_2$ of 98%, oxygen content could be inadequate. Conversely, patients with

high levels of Hb (e.g. some chronic respiratory patients) may have adequate oxygen content with very low $S_pO_2$.

Normal $S_pO_2$ on air is above 95%, so anything less than this should be investigated. Less than 92% is significant (in patients with no pre-existing respiratory disease) and oxygen therapy should be considered, but expect slightly lower values in elderly patients, heavy smokers and during sleep. Look for trends and report any deterioration (e.g. a consistent $S_pO_2$ of 90% may be less worrying in some cases than saturations that have suddenly dropped from 98% to 92%). Patients with reduced cardiac output should normally have $S_pO_2$ maintained above 94%. In the chronic respiratory patient hypoxaemia may not be significant until $S_pO_2$ drops below 80–85% owing to increased Hb.

### DOCUMENTATION

This should be recorded in the respiratory section of the assessment.

Record $S_pO_2$ measurement, the patient's position and any activity undertaken. Note inspired oxygen concentration during measurement and the type of oxygen delivery device, if used.

## 3.49 PUPILS (SEE ALSO 3.33 GLASGOW COMA SCACE)

### DEFINITION

Pupil size and reactivity (response to light) is important in neurological assessment. Changes may reflect pressure on the nerves of the eye (optic and oculomotor) or an increased pressure within the cranium (skull) or the effect of some drugs.

### PURPOSE

Pupillary assessment allows physiotherapists to monitor changes in a patient's status as this may require an urgent response, e.g. may indicate a neurological deterioration. This is often recorded alongside GCS (see 3.33 Glasgow Coma Scale) using a scale such as the one in Fig. 3.49.1.

### PROCEDURE

- To assess pupils you need a pen-torch.
- If the patient is sedated/asleep you will have to hold the eyelids open.
- Observe the pupils for size and shape.
- Briefly shine a light into the eyes, noting whether they react both when the light is shining and once taken away.

## ASSESSMENT TOOLS

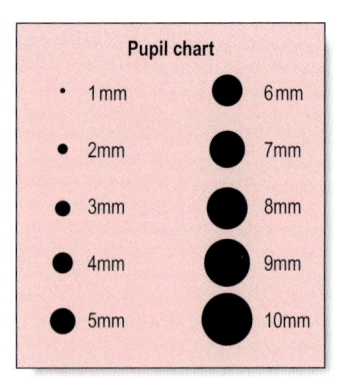

**Fig 3.49.1** Pupil size chart.

### FINDINGS
- Normal pupils will constrict to light; this is marked as '+' on the record sheet. If there is no reaction, it is marked as '–'.
- A slowed response can be described as sluggish and is marked as '+/–' or 's'.
- Normal pupil size is 2–3 mm. Fixed dilated pupils are a very poor sign and may indicate brain stem death. However, the drugs a patient is receiving may adversely affect pupil reaction. For example, the heavy sedative thiopentone can cause fixed dilated pupils, as can atrovent nebulizers if they get into the eye, and opiates (e.g. morphine) can cause pinpoint pupils. It is also important to know whether the person has any previous eye problems as this may distort the assessment, e.g. cataract surgery.

Any change in reaction should always be highlighted to senior colleagues, particularly fixed, sluggish or unequal responses as these may reflect an acute change in status requiring prompt action.

### DOCUMENTATION
Pupil size and reactivity should be recorded in the CNS section of your assessment. A normal pupillary response on assessment is often written as PEARL – or pupils equal and reactive to light. Any change in status since last review or during intervention should also be noted.

## 3.50 QUALITY OF LIFE QUESTIONNAIRES

### DEFINITION
There are a number of questionnaires and scales that have been designed to quantify the impact of respiratory disease on the patient's life.

## 3.50 Quality of life questionnaires

### PURPOSE
These are used mainly as outcome measures to test the effectiveness of medical and pharmacological treatments and other interventions such as pulmonary rehabilitation programmes. They aim to capture the patient's perspective and relate to their social participation. Outcome measures focus on body, structure and function. 'QoL' questionnaires relate to a patient's perspective and their social participation: they are more client-centred and potentially more relevant.

These questionnaires may also be used as a starting point when helping set patient goals for physiotherapy treatments.

### PROCEDURE
Choose the questionnaire that seems most appropriate for the patient or the one currently used by your department for audit. Some questionnaires are 'disease specific' whereas others are 'generic' to many diseases. Respiratory disease-specific questionnaires tend to focus on the problems that breathlessness causes in everyday life.

#### Some commonly seen questionnaires
- St Georges Respiratory Questionnaire for COPD (SGRQ-C)
- Pulmonary Functional Status and Dyspnoea Questionnaire (PFSDQ)
- Chronic Respiratory Disease Questionnaire (CRQ)
- Short Form Chronic Respiratory disease Questionnaire (SF CRQ)
- Short Form 36 (SF 36)
- Asthma Quality of Life questionnaire.

Questionnaires may be left with the patient to complete, or may be completed by an interviewer working with the patient. This option is particularly important for patients who are unable to read and write or who have cognitive problems and may need further prompting. Decide on the most appropriate option for your patient.

### FINDINGS
Most questionnaires have a standardized scoring scheme and information regarding the significance of the scores and what would constitute a clinically valid effect from treatment.

### DOCUMENTATION
Record time of completion and score. Note any issues affecting the patient such as a current infection or any emotional upset.

## OBTAINING THE QUESTIONNAIRES

- St Georges Respiratory Questionnaire (SGRQ-C). Available at: P.W. Jones, PhD FRCP, Professor of Respiratory Medicine, St George's University of London, Cranmer Terrace, London SW17 ORE, UK; Tel.: +44 (0) 20 8725 5371; http://www.healthstatus.sgul.ac.uk/SGRQ_download/SGRQ-C%20English%202008.pdf
- Pulmonary Function and Dyspnoea Questionnaire (PFSDQ). Available at: Ms S.C. Lareau, Pulmonary Clinical Nurse Specialist, Jerry L. Pettis Memorial Veterans Hospital, 11201 Benton Street, Loma Linda, CA 92357, USA; Email: lareau.suzanne@loma-linda.va. gov
- Chronic Respiratory Disease Questionnaire (CRDQ, CRQ). Available at: Jane Howe, Licensing Officer, Office of Research Contracts & Intellectual Property, McMaster University, GH 306G, 1280 Main Street, W. Hamilton, Ontario, Canada L8S 4L8; Email: orcip@mcmastr.ca
- Asthma Quality of Life Questionnaire. Available at: Qoltech, Professor Elizabeth Juniper/Mrs Jilly Styles, 20 Marcuse Fields, Bosham PO18 8NA, UK; http://www.qoltech.co.uk/obtaining.html
- SF 36, modified version. Available at: RAND Health Communications, 1776 Main Street, PO Box 2138, Santa Monica, CA 90407-2138, USA; http://www.rand.org/health/surveys_tools/mos/mos_core_36item_survey.html

## 3.51 RATING OF PERCEIVED EXERTION (RPE)

### DEFINITION
A numeric scale used to rate the level of effort (exertion) felt by the patient/participant during a particular exercise or activity.

### PURPOSE
Used during exercise testing to identify the patient's response at each stage as a supplement to, or instead of, HR. Also used to prescribe and monitor appropriate exercise intensity for patients participating in exercise programmes and as an outcome measure for research. It is particularly useful where HR response to exercise is not reliable, such as with patients on β-blocking drugs or people with respiratory limitations to exercise.

### PROCEDURE
Two scales are frequently used: Borg (original) RPE and Borg (revised) CR10. (These scales can also be adapted to rate breathlessness, see 3.8 Breathlessness measurement.) Table 3.51.1 summarizes both of these scales.

## 3.51 Rating of perceived exertion (RPE)

**Table 3.51.1 Borg RPE scale and Borg CR10 scale**

| Borg RPE scale | | Borg CR10 scale | |
|---|---|---|---|
| 6 | No exertion at all | 0 | Nothing at all |
| 7 | Very, very light | 0.3 | |
| 8 | | 0.5 | Extremely weak (just noticeable) |
| 9 | Very light | 1 | Very weak/light |
| 10 | | 1.5 | |
| 11 | Fairly light | 2 | Weak (light) |
| 12 | | 3 | Moderate |
| 13 | Somewhat hard | 3.5 | |
| 14 | | 4.5 | |
| 15 | Hard | 5.5 | |
| 16 | | 6.5 | |
| 17 | Very hard | 7.5 | |
| 18 | | 9 | |
| 19 | Extremely hard | 10 | Extremely strong, almost maximal |
| 20 | Maximal exertion | * maximal | |

Adapted from Borg Perception.

- Choose a scale and print in large font so it can easily be seen by the patient during the exercise.
- Ask the patient to familiarize themselves with the scale and then choose (call out or point to) the number that best describes the amount of 'effort' or 'exertion' they feel they are making during the exercise. They should focus on how heavy or strenuous the exercise feels overall rather than on any specific symptoms.
- This can be repeated at every level during an exercise test or during regular intervals (e.g. every minute).

### FINDINGS

This is a subjective measure of how the individual feels, and may vary from person to person, so ideally the RPE should be considered in conjunction with HR. There is normally good correlation between RPE and HR, so that, for most people, their HR will be approximately 10 times their RPE score (providing the original scale is used). If you have measured both during a test you could look to see whether this correlation was demonstrated. If not, your participant might be underestimating or overestimating the intensity of exercise and may need to be encouraged to work less hard or to work harder, depending on what is most appropriate for them. When prescribing exercise we normally encourage people to work at a 'moderate' to 'somewhat severe' intensity (12–14 on the RPE scale or 3–4 on the CR10 scale), so you can help your patient to 'learn' what constitutes an appropriate level by practising using this rating scale and giving them feedback.

## DOCUMENTATION

When recording, it is important to state which scale is being used and to record the RPE alongside the corresponding intensity of exercise/stage of exercise test.

## FURTHER READING

Borg, G., 2004. The Borg CR10 Scale. Borg Perception, Hässelby, Sweden. For information about scale construction, administration, etc., see Borg G., 1998. Borg's Perceived Exertion and Pain Scales. Human Kinetics, Champaign, IL. Scales and instructions can be obtained for a minor fee from Dr G. Borg. E-mail: borgperception@telia.com

Centres for Disease Control and Prevention, 2010. Physical Activity for Everyone. Available at: http://www.cdc.gov/physicalactivity/everyone/measuring/exertion.html

## 3.52 REFLEXES

### DEFINITION

An involuntary and nearly instantaneous muscle contraction in response to a stimulus, e.g. a tap by a patellar hammer. Reflexes are used to review various aspects of the patient's neurology.

### PURPOSE

Some reflexes that may be used in respiratory care are:

- *Reflexes to protect the airway*: coughs and sneezes are reflexes developed to protect the airway as a result of mechanical stimulation. Swallow is a complex reflex to protect the airway while eating or drinking (see 3.19 Cough assessment and 3.60 Swallow assessment).
- *Reflexes to review neurology*: reflex tests are used in a variety of clinical situations to form part of a wider assessment. This is often carried out alongside assessment of dermatomes, myotomes and muscle grading (see appropriate sections). If there is

## 3.52 Reflexes

muscle weakness, reflex testing aids in distinguishing between muscle wasting and neurological damage. This may be in the trauma patient or the neurologically impaired. The results may affect how the patient is managed at a later stage and changes in reflexes should be reported to the team. Some examples follow; this is by no means a comprehensive list and the reader is directed to other texts for more detail:
- Pupil reflex: used to check for brain stem function, often used if a patient shows signs of neurological deterioration (see 3.49 Pupils).
- Deep tendon reflexes (e.g. patella or knee-jerk reflex): used to check the integrity of the reflex arc and the nerve supply of the muscle being tested. This may form part of a comprehensive assessment in critical care.

### PROCEDURE
- Pupil reflex: see 3.49 Pupils for procedure and findings.
- Deep tendon reflexes: a gentle tap is applied to the tendon with a patella hammer; see Further reading for details of the procedure.
- Plantar reflex: a blunt instrument is drawn up the lateral border of the foot from heel to toe; see Further reading.

### FINDINGS
- Deep tendon reflexes: one side should be compared with the other.
- Plantar reflex: in health the great toe will flex. This response may be absent or the toe may extend in patients with upper motor nerve lesions or damage.

### DOCUMENTATION
- Deep tendon reflexes are described as 'normal, brisk, absent or slow'. Record whether right and left are the same.
- Plantar reflex is recorded as normal, absent or upgoing plantar. Record whether the right and left are the same.

### FURTHER READING
Day, R., Fox, J., Paul-Taylor, G., 2009. Neuro-musculoskeletal Clinical Testing: A Clinician's Guide. Churchill Livingstone, Edinburgh, UK.

Jones, K., 2011. Neurological Assessment: A Clinician's Guide. Churchill Livingstone, Edinburgh, UK.

## 3.53 RENAL FUNCTION (See under 3.6 BLOOD RESULTS and 3.31 FLUID BALANCE – pages 49 and 102)

## 3.54 RESPIRATORY PATTERN (SEE ALSO 3.55 RESPIRATORY RATE)

### DEFINITION
The term used by physiotherapists when referring to the observed movements and muscle activity in the thorax (ribs and sternum), shoulder girdle and abdomen during the cycles of inhalation and exhalation is often referred to as the respiratory pattern.

### PURPOSE
Observation and monitoring of breathing pattern provides information regarding the possible underlying respiratory disease and can, along with RR, also detect any change in a patient's condition (improvement or deterioration).

### PROCEDURE
- Assess alongside RR (see 3.55 Respiratory rate).
- Try to observe without drawing the patient's attention to their breathing as this is likely to cause it to change.
- If dignity and warmth allow, the patient should be undressed from the waist up.
- Observe from both the front and the side of the patient.
- Monitor the overall rise and fall of the chest wall and determine the degree of contribution from the upper chest area (ribs 1–7), the lower chest area (ribs 8–12) and the abdomen.
- Note the patient's posture and any movement of the shoulder girdle (e.g. protraction, elevation).
- Observe the neck and shoulders for signs of muscle activity in the accessory muscles, e.g. sternomastoid, scalenes or pectoralis major during inspiration.
- Observe and palpate the abdomen for any signs of abdominal muscle activity during expiration.
- Observe the head and face for signs of effort, nostril flaring or head bobbing movement.
- Monitor breathing pattern during resting breathing and also during deep breathing manoeuvres.
- During assessment and treatment any changes in breathing pattern can be observed, e.g. change in breathing pattern in response to exercise or in response to nasopharyngeal suction.

## 3.54 Respiratory pattern

### FINDINGS
See Table 3.54.1.

**Table 3.54.1 Breathing pattern definitions**

| Breathing pattern | Definition/description |
|---|---|
| Tachypnoea | See 3.55 Respiratory rate |
| Bradypnoea | See 3.55 Respiratory rate |
| Apnoea | Total cessation of breathing for greater than 10 seconds |
| Hypopnoea | Term used to describe shallow breathing (<50% of normal) for greater than 10 seconds |
| Hypoventilation | Reduced total ventilation (rate × tidal volume). Most commonly seen with sedation or opiate analgesia. Normally causes a rise in arterial carbon dioxide ($P_aCO_2$) |
| Hyperventilation | Increased total ventilation (rate × tidal volume). Most commonly seen with anxiety, pain or hyperventilation syndrome. Normally causes a reduction in arterial carbon dioxide ($P_aCO_2$) |
| Pursed lip breathing | The patient will be seen to oppose their lips during expiration in order to maintain pressure within the thorax and prevent the smaller airways from collapsing (also known as intrinsic PEEP). This is often seen in patients with severe COPD or other airways diseases |
| Accessory muscle use | Accessory muscles in the neck or shoulder region suggest increased work of breathing that may be related to lung hyperinflation and chronic obstructive disease |
| Apical breathing | When respiratory movement is mainly seen in the upper chest and shoulder area this may be associated with increased respiratory effort and/or anxiety or stress |
| Diaphragmatic or lower chest breathing | When respiratory movements mainly occur in the lower chest region or abdomen, this may be associated with a more relaxed and efficient pattern with less effort involved |
| Localized hyperinflation | May signify a pneumothorax (check breath sounds (see 3.3 Auscultation)) |

*(Continued)*

## ASSESSMENT TOOLS

**Table 3.54.1  Breathing pattern definitions—cont'd**

| Breathing pattern | Definition/description |
|---|---|
| Reduced expansion or shallow breathing | May suggest restrictive problems such as fibrosing lung disease, muscle weakness or reduced movement due to abdominal distension. Unilateral reduced movement may be due to atelectasis, consolidation or localized fibrosis |
| Increased respiratory movement | At rest suggests increased minute volume. The patient may be hyperventilating (overbreathing), or there may be increased demand for respiration due to infection or injury |
| Cheyne–Stokes respiration | Irregular breathing with cycles consisting of a few relatively deep breaths followed by a period of progressively shallower breaths (sometimes to the point of apnoea), and then a gradual return to deeper breaths. This is often associated with heart failure, severe neurological disturbances or drugs (e.g. narcotics) |
| Kussmaul's respiration | Rapid, deep breathing with high minute ventilation (rate × tidal volume). Commonly seen in patients with metabolic acidosis |
| Ataxic breathing | Consists of haphazard, uncoordinated deep and shallow breathing. This may be found in patients with cerebellar disease |
| Apneustic breathing | Characterized by prolonged inspiration, and is usually the result of brain damage |

### DOCUMENTATION

The respiratory or breathing pattern should be recorded in the respiratory section of your objective assessment alongside RR. Any recent changes in breathing pattern should also be recorded especially if there has been a noticeable increase or decrease in the rate, or change in pattern of exhalation and inhalation. Any changes in breathing pattern when undergoing physiotherapy should be documented, as well as the time taken for the breathing pattern to return to baseline and whether any additional treatment was required to allow the pattern to return to baseline.

## 3.55 RESPIRATORY RATE (RR)

### DEFINITION
RR is the number of breaths (inhalation and exhalation) taken in 1 minute. It is usually determined by counting the number of times the chest rises or falls per minute, although it may be monitored by a spirometer or capnometer.

### PURPOSE
A patient's RR is one of the most important clinical assessments as it can give a clear indication of the patient's clinical condition.

> **Top tip!**
> RR is often the first sign of any improvement or deterioration in the patient's condition.

A raised RR is a strong and specific predictor of serious adverse events such as cardiac arrest and unplanned ITU admission. An adult with a RR of over 20 breaths per minute at rest is probably unwell, and an adult with a RR of over 24 breaths per minute at rest is likely to be critically ill.

### PROCEDURE
- Assess alongside respiratory pattern (see 3.54 Respiratory pattern).
- Try to observe without drawing the patient's attention to their breathing as this is likely to cause it to change.
- Count the number of breaths taken during 1 minute. (Counting for only 15 seconds and multiplying by 4 or any other similar technique is not an accurate measure.)
- Non-invasive monitoring equipment may not be accurate for calculating RR.

### FINDINGS
- The normal range is 12–16 breaths per minute.
- It is normal for RR to rise during exercise, excitement, pain and fever. It declines during relaxation and sleep.
- Tachypnoea is defined as a RR of greater than 20 breaths per minute, whereas bradypnoea is defined as a RR of less than 10 breaths per minute.
- Respiratory apnoea occurs when no breaths are taken or the chest fails to rise or fall. Prolonged apnoea will result in a respiratory arrest and is a medical emergency.

A patient's RR is a key indicator as to the stability of a patient to undergo physiotherapy treatment. As previously mentioned, it is normal for RR to rise during exercise (including walking) or many physiotherapy treatments (e.g. manual techniques or suction). The degree of rise will be dependent on the patient's exertion. In the absence of illness, this RR will return to normal within a few minutes of ceasing the activity.

Tachypnoea (high breathing rate) can be seen in any form of lung disease and is associated with an increase in work of breathing due to increased turbulence in the airways. Tachypnoea can lead to respiratory alkalosis as a result of a reduction in partial pressure of carbon dioxide ($P_aCO_2$). It may also occur with metabolic acidosis when the respiratory system is attempting to compensate for a metabolic failure.

Bradypnoea (low breathing rate) is a relatively uncommon finding, and is usually due to CNS depression by narcotics, sedatives (e.g. morphine) or trauma (e.g. head injury or brain stem infarct). This often leads to an increase in $P_aCO_2$ and therefore leads to respiratory acidosis (see 3.1 Arterial blood gases). Bradypnoea may also be seen in severe chronic bronchitis, when the patient may breathe more slowly to reduce their work of breathing.

### DOCUMENTATION
The RR should be recorded when documenting a patient's vital signs alongside respiratory pattern. Any recent changes in RR should also be recorded, especially if there has been a noticeable increase or decrease in the rate. Any changes in RR when undergoing physiotherapy should be documented, as well as the time taken for RR to return to baseline and whether any additional treatment was required to allow the RR to return to baseline.

## 3.56 RESUSCITATION STATUS

### DEFINITION
The medical team may categorize the patient's status according to whether or not they should be given resuscitation (basic life support). This is commonly shortened to 'resus status'. It should also be recorded what active treatments are to be provided such as medication (e.g. antibiotics), NG feeding or suction.

### PURPOSE
Physiotherapists must understand the limitations of treatment and thus adjust their approach accordingly.

Appendix 2

**Do Not Attempt Cardiopulmonary Resuscitation Order**

(This form to be kept in the front of the medical records)

| Patient Details | | |
|---|---|---|
| Address label | Admission Date | -------------- |
| | Hospital | -------------- |
| | Ward | -------------- |

**Reason for DNAR order**

- ☐ Patient has refused CPR
- ☐ Patient is clearly in the terminal phase of illness
- ☐ The burdens of treatment outweigh the benefits

**This decision must be documented in writing below**

**Communication with patient/family:**

Date of Decision: ____________ Decision by: ____________

Consultant/GP (print)

| | | |
|---|---|---|
| Consultant/GP informed of decision: | Yes | No |
| Primary Nurse/Senior nursing staff informed:<br>Name: | Yes | No |

Signature: ____________ Review Date: ________ by ________

Consultant/GP ________ by ________

________ by ________

________ by ________

Interim Signature:* ____________ ________ by ________

Registered Medical Practitioner

*If consultant/GP has not been contacted at the time of decision

**Fig 3.56.1** Example resuscitation form.
Used with permission from Cardiff and Vale University Health Board

## *PROCEDURE*

Although physiotherapists may be asked their opinion with regard to resuscitation, it is only a senior doctor (generally senior registrar or consultant) who can document a 'not for resuscitation' order.

Commonly used terms are:

- Do not attempt resuscitation (DNAR)
- Not for resuscitation (NFR)

- Tender loving care (TLC): for supportive care or just to keep comfortable (no other medical interventions); at this point, many hospitals will use an end-of-life pathway.

### FINDINGS

If a patient is not for resuscitation or there are limitations of care in place, this should be clearly marked at the front of their notes on a resuscitation form (Fig. 3.56.1). If there is no comment on resuscitation status it should always be assumed that the patient is for full active care.

### DOCUMENTATION

A patient's resuscitation status (and if it changes) should be highlighted clearly in your physiotherapy database.

## 3.57 SEDATION/AGITATION SCORE (SEE ALSO 3.39 LEVEL OF CONSCIOUSNESS)

### DEFINITION

A scale used to assess sedation and agitation levels in hospital patients – especially critical care areas.

### PURPOSE

Sedation is used to allow good management of pain, anxiety and sleep. This enables patients to tolerate the hospital environment (be it the ward or critical care) and also the procedures that are required for their management and treatment.

In a critically ill patient, agitation, confusion, or both can result from the original medical condition or from medical complications, or can be the consequence of treatment or the environment. Critical care patients may be agitated, confused, uncomfortable or suffering from critical care delirium. This may affect how they interact with those around them or their ability to participate in treatment.

### PROCEDURE

The patient is scored against set criteria, which will depend upon the scale being used. This is a subjective scale and two common examples are reflected in Table 3.57.1.

## 3.57 Sedation/agitation score

**Table 3.57.1 Sedation scores**

| Ramsay sedation score | Riker Sedation–Agitation Scale |
|---|---|
| 1. Patient is anxious and agitated or restless, or both | 7. Dangerous agitation: pulling at ETT, trying to remove catheters, climbing over bedrail, striking at staff, thrashing side-to-side |
| 2. Patient is cooperative, oriented and tranquil | 6. Very agitated: requiring restraint and frequent verbal reminding of limits, biting ETT |
| 3. Patient responds to commands only | 5. Agitated: anxious or physically agitated, calms to verbal instructions |
| 4. Patient exhibits brisk response to light glabellar tap or loud auditory stimulus | 4. Calm and cooperative: calm, easily arousable, follows commands |
| 5. Patient exhibits a sluggish response to light glabellar tap or loud auditory stimulus | 3. Sedated: difficult to arouse but awakens to verbal stimuli or gentle shaking, follows simple commands but drifts off again |
| 6. Patient exhibits no response | 2. Very sedated: arouses to physical stimuli but does not communicate or follow commands, may move spontaneously |
|  | 1. Unarousable: minimal or no response to noxious stimuli |

### FINDINGS

Changes in score may reflect the level of sedation that the patient requires. If there has been no change in medication and the score deteriorates, this may be due to worsening in the patient's condition. As can be seen from the two common examples, there are very different interpretations for each numbered value, e.g. '6' can mean agitated or unresponsive! It is, therefore, very important to note which scale you are using. Remember that physiotherapy intervention can be a stimulus and that sedation score may change with treatment.

### DOCUMENTATION

The sedation score should be noted in the CNS section of your assessment along with any change in status during your intervention.

## FURTHER READING

Ramsay, M.A., Savege, T.M., Simpson, B.R., Goodwin, R., 1974. Controlled sedation with alphaxalone-alphadolone. Br. Med. J. 2, 656–9.

Riker, R., Pickard, J., Fraser, G., 1999. Prospective evaluation of the Sedation-Agitation Scale for adult critically ill patients. Crit. Care Med. 27, 1325–9.

## 3.58 SPUTUM ASSESSMENT

### DEFINITION
A subjective review of the volume and nature of secretions cleared by the patient.

### PURPOSE
There are many patients who clear sputum as a matter of course (e.g. COPD or bronchiectatic patients). An early sign of an exacerbation can be a change in the nature or volume of the sputum they produce. Changes in sputum may also indicate an improvement or deterioration in patients with acute respiratory infection and the patient's response to treatment.

### PROCEDURE
This information would be gained either in discussion with the patient or by examining what the patient is expectorating

### FINDINGS
#### Sputum volume
An estimate of the volume can be made in discussion with the patient. This tends to be done in terms which the patient can understand, either in teaspoon or cups. A teaspoon has the volume of 5 ml. Has there been a change in the volume of sputum that the patient is producing?

Within critical care many units have a scale as to the volume cleared on suction:

- 1 = minimal (barely in the suction catheter)
- 2 = moderate (gets to the head of the suction catheter)
- 3 = copious (gets beyond catheter into the suction tubing).

#### Colour
Has there been a change in the colour of the sputum being produced? The colour is an indication of the clinical pathology, for example:

- white = minimal infection
- yellow or green = infection

- red = haemoptysis (fresh blood)
- brown = previous haemoptysis or lung tissue damage (old blood).

Large volumes of fresh blood must be reported to the medical team immediately.

Within critical care many units will use a code to describe colour of sputum:

- M = mucoid (clear secretions)
- P = purulent (this means coloured sputum)
- MP = mucopurulent (mixture of M and P)
- B = bloodstained (this may mean flecks of blood or plugs).

### Viscosity (rheology) or ease of expectoration

The rheology can be formally measured, but this is not often the case in clinical practice. Simple observation of the sputum will give an indication of the viscosity. Does the sputum move in the pot? If not, it is viscous. Does the patient find it easy to clear? Is it difficult to get the sputum up a suction catheter? Again, these would indicate that the sputum was more viscous and so harder to clear.

### Smell

Anaerobic bacteria or fungal infections may well produce an offensive smell, which should be documented.

### Taste

There is no suggestion at this point that you should taste the sputum! However, as in terms of smell, there may be occasions when the patient reports an unpleasant taste in their mouth.

## DOCUMENTATION

Document sputum production under the headings suggested above in the respiratory section of your assessment and also as an outcome of treatment.

For example:

- 'Normally clears clear yellow sputum easily'
- 'Large volumes of sticky green sputum cleared on suction (3MP)'.

## 3.59 SURGICAL INCISIONS

### DEFINITION

The site of entry or wound for an operative procedure.

## ASSESSMENT TOOLS

### PURPOSE
Knowledge of incision sites allows physiotherapists to identify patients who are at high risk of postoperative pulmonary complications. Although some operations have a relatively small incision they can have a huge impact on respiratory function!

### PROCEDURE
An example of common incision sites is shown in Fig. 3.59.1.

### FINDINGS
Thoracic and high abdominal incisions will have the greatest impact on the respiratory system. Alongside incision site, pain management should also be considered (see 3.44 Pain score) as both these factors will affect the patient's ability to participate in treatment. Low abdominal and pelvic incisions have a lower risk of pulmonary complications but a higher risk of DVT.

### DOCUMENTATION
When documenting operation notes in your physiotherapy notes, you should include the incision site and findings of the surgery.

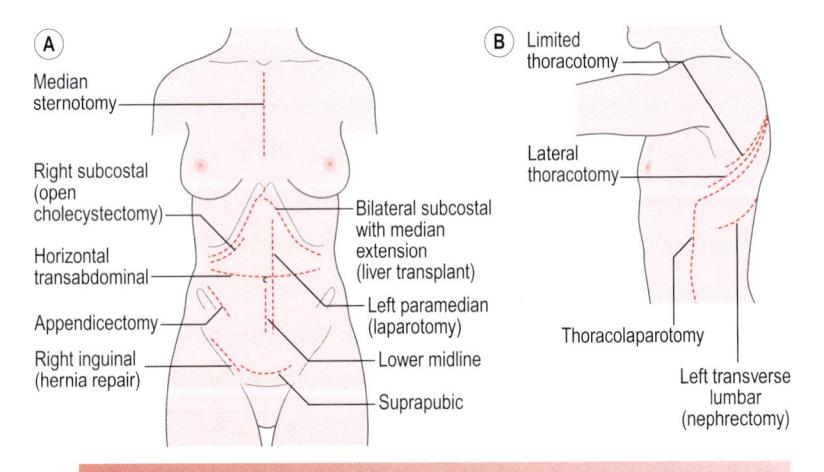

**Fig 3.59.1** (A,B) Surgical incisions.
Reproduced with kind permission from Pryor JA, Prasad SA. 2008 Physiotherapy for Respiratory and Cardiac Problems, 4th Edn. Edinburgh, UK: Churchill Livingstone.

## 3.60 SWALLOW ASSESSMENT

### DEFINITION

An evaluation of a patient's bulbar function (ability to swallow) to ascertain whether a patient is likely to aspirate (food or fluid going into the respiratory tract).

### PURPOSE

Swallowing is a combination of several phases and disruption of any one of these can affect safe swallowing. Patients with oropharyngeal muscle weakness, swelling or loss of airway protective reflexes are at risk of aspiration. At-risk patients include those with acute neurological conditions (such as stroke and head trauma) or chronic neurological diseases (such as motor neurone disease and dementia) and following head and neck surgery. Patients with a tracheostomy are also at greater risk of aspiration. Physiotherapists need to be aware of patients with swallowing difficulties as they are also likely to have problems with secretion management and sputum clearance. It is also important to know whether a patient has been designated as nil by mouth (NBM) because of problems with swallowing.

### PROCEDURE

A formal swallow assessment should only be carried out by clinical staff with appropriate training, i.e. a speech and language therapist.

### FINDINGS

Patients who are unable to swallow safely will be designated as NBM. Physiotherapists often work closely with speech and language therapists, and, once a patient is recommenced on an oral intake, we may be asked to keep a close eye on respiratory function. Those patients who are NBM are often very dry, and this can have an effect on the viscosity (thickness) of secretions.

### DOCUMENTATION

If a patient has a compromised swallow this should be documented in the database of your notes and any change in function clearly marked on subsequent assessments.

## 3.61 TPR (TEMPERATURE, PULSE AND RESPIRATION) CHART

### DEFINITION
A record of repeated measurements of body temperature, pulse, RR and blood pressure in a graphical format (additional information may include fluid balance, blood results, pain or sedation scores and early warning scores) (Fig. 3.61.1).

### PURPOSE
Used for monitoring patients in hospital wards or those receiving frequent nursing at home. Identifies any trends or patterns that indicate the patient's health status (e.g. stable, variable, recovering or deteriorating). Helps determine suitability for physiotherapy treatment. It has particular importance in the early identification of the deteriorating patient at risk of critical illness or death.

### PROCEDURE
Although normally a nursing procedure, physiotherapists may be required to take these measurements and/or fill in the chart, e.g. when visiting patients as part of a 'hospital at home' scheme or when attending a patient who appears acutely unwell.

#### Body temperature
- Do not measure within 1 hour of the patient having a bath or vigorous exercise.
- Wait 20 minutes before measuring after a hot or cold drink (if using the mouth).
- Electronic thermometers can be used at the mouth, axilla, ear or rectum and give a digital display. Follow the instructions for individual devices.
- Clean the thermometer with an alcohol wipe or as directed by infection control:
  - Mouth: place under the tongue and close the mouth. Leave it in place for 3 minutes (or until it beeps).
  - Axilla: place the thermometer in the armpit, with the arm pressed against the body for 5 minutes before reading.
  - Ear: place a new cover over the probe, place the probe in the ear and press the start/measure key. A digital readout will appear when the machine beeps (Fig. 3.61.2).
- Plastic strip thermometers change colour to indicate temperature. Place the strip on the forehead and read it after 1 minute while the strip is in place.

## 3.61 TPR (temperature, pulse and respiration) chart

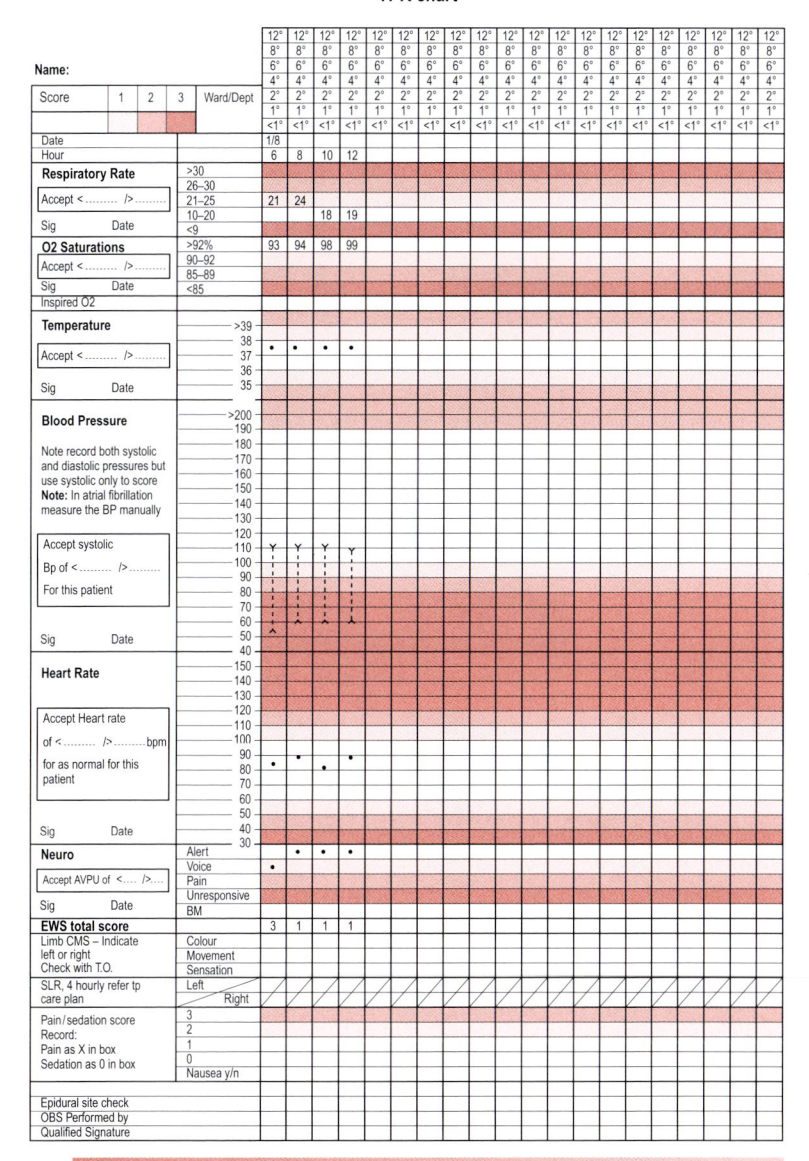

**Fig 3.61.1** Temperature pulse and respiratory rate chart (also known as a TPR or vital signs chart). Different hospitals use alternative charting systems. Of note this chart includes both early warning and pain scores.
Used with permission from Cardiff and Vale University Health Board

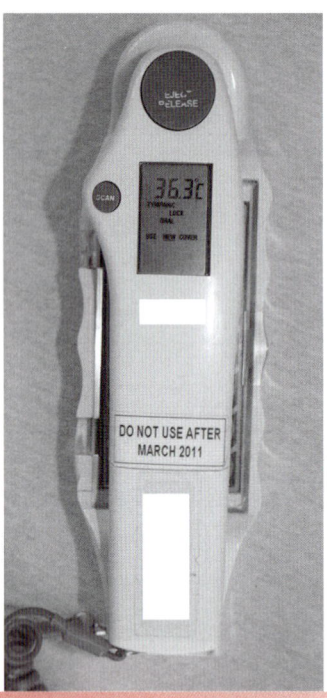

**Fig 3.61.2** Tympanic (ear) thermometer.

## *Pulse (HR)*
- Pulse may be taken manually or using automated machines alongside BP measurements. For procedure, see 3.34 Heart rate.

## *Respiration*
- For procedure, see 3.55 Respiratory rate.

> **Top tip!**
> RR is often an early marker of deterioration and, if not marked on the chart, you should assess for yourself!

## *Blood pressure*
- For procedure, see 3.5 Blood pressure.

## FINDINGS
### Body temperature
- Temperature may vary, so it is important to find out what is normal for the patient. It is normally highest in the evening and can be influenced by room temperature and humidity.

## 3.61 TPR (temperature, pulse and respiration) chart

**Table 3.61.1  Normal temperature ranges**

| Ear | 35.7–38.0°C | 96.4–100.4°F |
|---|---|---|
| Oral | 36.5–37.5°C | 95.9–99.5°F |
| Axillary (armpit) | 34.7–37.2°C | 94.5–99.1°F |

May be raised by anxiety, pain, physical activity, warm clothing, after eating or by the actions of some drugs. Normal ranges are summarized in Table 3.61.1.

- Pyrexia (fever) may be diagnosed when temperature increases to more than 1°C above the patient's normal, suggesting an infection which has caused the body's thermal regulatory mechanism to 'reset' to a higher level.
- Fever may be intermittent or continuous so it is important to look for trends.

> **Top tip!**
> After surgery, a reflex pyrexia (when body temperature gradually rises and falls within 24 hours of surgery) is common and does not necessarily imply infection.

- Hyperpyrexia: fever with an extreme elevation of temperature above or equal to 41.5°C (106.7°F). Requires immediate medical attention as it constitutes a medical emergency and may be life threatening.
- Hypothermia is defined as a drop in body temperature below 35°C (95°F).

### Pulse, BP and RR

- Look for trends.
- A general increase over time in all three measurements (above normal levels) suggests increased sympathetic activity which may be linked to worsening pathology and/or anxiety/stress. This could eventually lead to fatigue and needs to be highlighted to the medical team. It may also affect the patient's ability to tolerate physiotherapy or any increase in activity levels.
- An increase in pulse rate seen in combination with a drop in BP is a potentially serious sign of impending circulatory shock and should be highlighted to the medical team (see Documentation below).

## ASSESSMENT TOOLS

- A trend towards decreasing values below normal limits may be due to impaired cerebral function and loss of sympathetic outflow requiring immediate medical intervention.
- A grossly raised BP compared with HR in a patient with a spinal injury above T6 can be a sign of autonomic dysreflexia and should be treated as a medical emergency.

> **Top tip!**
> If you are unsure about unusual measurements on a TPR chart, it is important to highlight your concerns to a senior – you may be the first person to have identified a problem.

### DOCUMENTATION

- These charts vary so find out what is required for your specific chart.
- Ensure recordings are entered in alignment with the appropriate date and time.
- Use the appropriate 'scale' – there are normally separate scales for temperature, HR and BP together, and respiration (Fig. 3.61.1).
- Temperature, HR and respiration are usually recorded with a dot, but blood pressure is recorded with a 'v' shape at the top representing systolic pressure, an inverted 'v' below representing diastolic pressure and a dotted line is drawn between the two (Fig. 3.61.1).

> **Top tip!**
> Unlike Fig 3.61.1 some charts have HR and BP on the same scale. Here, the 'v' at the top of the BP column (systolic pressure reading) looks a bit like a seagull and the dot for the pulse represents the seagull's dropping. You would expect to see the dropping below the bird! If the dropping is above the bird, this is an indication of physiological compromise which needs addressing promptly. (see 3.5 Blood pressure).

## 3.62 VENTILATION–PERFUSION (V/Q) MATCHING

### DEFINITION

The ratio between ventilation (V) and perfusion (Q) demonstrates the degree of 'matching' between the distribution of ventilation in the lungs and the distribution of the blood flow. This is important because the better the two are matched, the better the gas exchange.

## 3.62 Ventilation–perfusion (V/Q) matching

### PURPOSE

It is useful for the physiotherapist to identify when a lung, lobe or segment is well ventilated but not well perfused (or perfused but not well ventilated) because it may be possible to improve ventilation and/or perfusion through a change of position (see Findings).

### PROCEDURE

Physiotherapists are not involved in the formal assessment of ventilation and perfusion matching. This can be assessed in the radiology department using a ventilation–perfusion scan or CTPA (see 3.14 Chest imaging (including chest radiographs)). However, it is useful for us to be aware of the principles of ventilation and perfusion matching.

Gas exchange can be monitored by oxygen saturations, ABGs and RR (see relevant sections). If a patient is hypoxaemic, or very breathless, it is useful to consider whether a change in the patient's body position might improve oxygenation or breathlessness.

### FINDINGS
#### Key terms

- Shunt: an area with no ventilation – so can be viewed as wasted perfusion.
- Dead space: an area with no perfusion – so could be viewed as wasted ventilation.

#### Normal lungs (adults)

In health, in the upright position, blood flow is preferentially distributed to the dependent areas of the lungs, as is the ventilation (e.g. in standing this would be the bases of the lungs). This results in a good match of the ventilation and perfusion. Less effective ventilation and perfusion occurs in the non-dependent areas of the lung (e.g. in standing this would be the apices). Thus, position affects ventilation and perfusion. However, there are pathologies in which the two may not match as well and this can lead to hypoxaemia or increased work of breathing.

A mismatch could be caused by a defect in perfusion, e.g. a pulmonary embolus, which will lead to dead space. Alternatively, it could be due to a defect in ventilation, such as atelectasis or consolidation in one lung (or in one or more lobe or segment, e.g. a lobar pneumonia). This will lead to a shunt.

As physiotherapists we may be able to improve ventilation to a lung, or lobe, through positioning, breathing techniques or positive pressure devices. The therapist can also affect the perfusion to the lungs. Blood flow is affected by gravity, so perfusion of the lungs can be influenced by posture .For example, a patient with a right lower lobe pneumonia will have a V/Q mismatch because of a lack of ventilation in that area. Positioning the patient in left side lying will allow more perfusion to the well-ventilated left lung. This position may also aid drainage of secretions from the right lower lobe. See Further reading.

If this patient is on a ventilator (i.e. positive pressure) the V/Q matching will change. Perfusion will remain the same because of gravity, but the area of best ventilation will be in the opposite direction of the self-ventilating adult (this is because positive pressure takes the path of least resistance). In this situation, positioning a patient with a right lower lobe pneumonia in left side lying will increase perfusion to the left lung but will reduce its ventilation. This may cause a detrimental effect on the patient's blood gases (see section 3.1 Arterial blood gases). See also Further reading.

## DOCUMENTATION

Record the posture in which the patient has optimal respiratory status in terms of saturations and RR. If the patient is saturating better in one position, this should be noted within your documentation. Similarly, if they have a tendency to desaturate in a particular position this should be noted.

## FURTHER READING

West, J.B., 2008. Respiratory Physiology: The Essentials, 8th edn. Lippincott, Williams and Wilkins, Baltimore, MD.

## 3.63 VENTILATOR OBSERVATIONS

### DEFINITION

Ventilator observations are the measurements of different ventilation parameters that are shown on the ventilator display, including measures such as the type of ventilation mode, tidal volume, minute volume and RR.

### PURPOSE

It is important for the physiotherapist to distinguish between patients for whom the ventilator is completely controlling the breathing pattern (controlled modes of ventilation/fully ventilated, e.g. CMV) and those where the ventilator is simply supporting the patient's own breathing (supported modes of ventilation, e.g. CPAP and pressure support). This may affect what you can do; for example, if a patient is fully ventilated they cannot breathe if disconnected from a ventilator and will be unable to participate in treatment. However, if a patient is on a supported mode, it may be possible for you to work with them to affect their breathing, e.g. using active cycle of breathing technique. The reader is directed towards the Findings and Further reading sections.

Ventilation observations can be used as an objective marker, e.g. lung compliance may increase following physiotherapy and the pressure required to ventilate the patient may be reduced.

Some physiotherapists alter ventilator settings as part of their role, e.g. for weaning purposes or in some cases to set up and manage NIV. This is only appropriate for senior staff with appropriate training!

## *PROCEDURE*

This is a straightforward process as most ventilators used in an acute setting, both invasive and non-invasive, have digital displays, and some have digital readings and graphs of pressure tracings. Therefore, it is simple to read off the volumes delivered and the pressures achieved. Find out by asking nursing staff and observing.

Additionally, for patients on ventilators at home, there are software packages which allow healthcare professionals to download information to study how the ventilator is used for further information.

## *FINDINGS*

Know your ventilator! Different manufacturers use slightly different terminology. So ensure that you are being consistent with the machine your patient is on. Within this text generic terms will be used (Table 3.63.1).

The efficacy of ventilation should be viewed in conjunction with other clinical findings, such as the ABGs. Is the level of ventilation adequate for this patient? The ventilator parameters may need to be altered. However, it is not the role of the inexperienced physiotherapist to do this!

Modes of ventilation broadly fall into one of three categories: control modes in which the ventilator is completely controlling the breathing pattern of the patient such as controlled mandatory ventilation (CMV); support modes in which the ventilator is helping the patient to breathe, such as pressure support (PS); or transitional modes in which the ventilator will allow patients to

## ASSESSMENT TOOLS

| Table 3.63.1 | Ventilator terminology |
|---|---|
| CMV | Continuous mandatory ventilation: a form of ventilation that completely controls the breathing pattern of the patient |
| SIMV | Synchronized intermittent mandatory ventilation: ventilation that provides mandatory breaths of a set rate and volume while attempting to synchronize with the patient's spontaneous breathing pattern |
| PS or ASB | Pressure support or assisted spontaneous breathing: a support mode that provides pressure support to a patient's own spontaneous breathing |
| PEEP or CPAP | Positive end-expiratory pressure or continuous positive airways pressure: assists to overcome the resistance of the ETT and to splint the airways open to aid oxygenation |
| Volume regulation | Delivery of the gas to the patient is regulated according to a prescribed volume (measured in ml) |
| Pressure regulation | Delivery of the gas to the patient is regulated according to a prescribed pressure (measured in $cmH_2O$) |
| NIV | Non-invasive ventilation: a form of respiratory support delivered without an ETT via a mask applied over the face |

breathe by themselves; however, if they do not breathe adequately, the machine will take over. An example of this would be synchronized intermittent mandatory ventilation (SIMV). Another classification of ventilation is dependent on how the desired volume is achieved. This can be performed in two ways: either by setting a volume or by setting pressures.

Having established the patient on respiratory support, the obvious questions to ask are: Is the patient adequately supported? Are adequate tidal volumes being achieved? What pressures are being delivered?

### DOCUMENTATION

In part this is determined by the ventilator make. Different manufacturers will have produced minor variations on ventilator modes and so the documentation will be specific to that machine. The minimum should include:

- mode of ventilation (e.g. SIMV)
- amount of oxygen being delivered, and oxygen saturations
- tidal volumes (set versus delivered in volume control modes)
- RR (both set and measured)
- pressures (e.g. pressure control, pressure support and PEEP).

For example, 'SIMV via ETT, TV 450 ml, set rate 14 breaths per minute (nil spont), PEEP 5, PS 8, $F_iO_2$ 0.40, $S_pO_2$ 98%'.

This tells you that the patient is on SIMV via an endotracheal tube. They have a set tidal volume and, as there are no spontaneous breaths, the machine is doing all the work. They are on low levels of PEEP (to splint open the airways) and although they have a pressure support set they are not using it as they are not breathing for themselves.

### FURTHER READING

Bersten, A., Soni, N., 2008. Oh's Intensive Care Manual, 6th edn. Butterworth-Heinemann, Edinburgh, UK.

http://emedicine.medscape.com/article/810126-overview

http://www.ccmtutorials.com

Simonds, A.K., 2007. Non-Invasive Respiratory Support: A Practical Handbook, 3rd edn. Hodder Arnold, London, UK.

Singer, M., Webb, A., 2009. Oxford Handbook of Critical Care. Oxford University Press, Oxford, UK.

## 3.64 WORK OF BREATHING

### DEFINITION

Work of breathing is the observed results of increasing load on the respiratory muscles. This is closely linked to dyspnoea, the subjective experience of breathing discomfort and breathlessness. Patients with increased work of breathing will undoubtedly feel breathless (see also 3.8 Breathlessness (dyspnoea) scales).

### PURPOSE

Physiotherapists need to be able to recognize patients with an increased work of breathing because, if the load applied to the respiratory muscles is increased steadily, they will eventually reach a point when they can no longer cope owing to fatigue. As this occurs the patient slips into respiratory failure. Recognizing and avoiding this will allow early intervention and treatment of the underlying problem.

### PROCEDURE

> **Top tip!**
> How does your patient look? If they look like they have just finished a workout, but are sat in bed, distressed and uncomfortable, this is a warning sign – time to act.

Work of breathing can be measured objectively using invasive techniques but these are usually reserved for research work. Clinically, this tends to be the result of observations.

## Look

- The RR will increase as the work of breathing increases. However, if the muscles then become fatigued, the RR will fall – at this point the patient is critically ill (see 3.55 Respiratory rate).
- Respiratory pattern: look for the use of accessory muscles (scaleni, sternocleidomastoid and the upper fibres of trapezius). A paradoxical (reciprocal) breathing pattern (in which the abdomen is drawn in as the patient inhales) and pursed lipped breathing are signs of increased work of breathing (see 3.54 Respiratory pattern).
- It is also worth looking at ABGs if they are available (see 3.1 Arterial blood gases) as type 1 respiratory failure transforming to type 2 respiratory failure may be observable. This would indicate that the patient is fatiguing.

## Listen

- Ask yourself the following: on auscultation are there adequate breath sounds and is there adequate ventilation? If not, this may be due to fatigue. Does the breathing sound laboured?

## Feel

- When palpating for expansion, is it equal (see 3.45 Palpation)?

## FINDINGS

The observed work of breathing combines all these measures. It should be discussed with supervisors, who can guide you and link your theory to observation in practice.

Remember:

- Respiratory muscle strength: normal muscles cannot cope with an increase in load and will eventually fail. Initially, accessory muscles will be used to compensate. In some pathologies, this can occur even during normal ventilation. For example, patients with motor neurone disease, in which respiratory muscles are becoming progressively weaker and the patient eventually slips into respiratory failure.
- Load: the workload includes the chest wall itself, lung compliance and airways resistance.
- Chest wall: a heavy or stiff chest wall will result in the respiratory muscles needing to work harder. This occurs in restrictive disorders such as obesity and kyphoscoliosis.

- Lung compliance (stiffness of the lungs or the ability of the lungs to respond to stretch): stiffer lungs are harder to move. This occurs in progressive fibrotic lung disease, or acute conditions such as acute respiratory distress syndrome.
- Resistance of the airways: air flow obstruction will also result in an increase on the load of the respiratory muscle. This occurs in diseases such as asthma and COPD.

### *DOCUMENTATION*

Increased work of breathing can form part of a problem list of the assessment. It can also be documented under observation, e.g. 'patient has increased work of breathing – use of accessories and pursed lip breathing'.

Changes in work of breathing must also be documented as part of a systematic assessment or as part of a treatment analysis.

**CHAPTER**

# Case scenarios

**4**

4.1 Introduction   173
4.2 Case Scenarios   173

4.3 Suggested Answers   179

## 4.1 INTRODUCTION

The following scenarios portray real situations that are not uncommon in clinical practice. Working through them will allow you to pull together the information covered in this book in a problem-solving manner.

For each of the scenarios consider:

- the type of assessment you would undertake (e.g. systems based, functional, social)
- what your assessment aims and priorities would be
- the significance of your assessment findings.

Suggested solutions are provided at the end of this chapter, with explanations to guide your clinical reasoning. These solutions are not all-encompassing, so other ideas may be worth pursuing, e.g. you could discuss your ideas with your supervisor or mentor. You may need to look back at individual assessment tools for further information.

## 4.2 CASE SCENARIOS

### SURGICAL EXAMPLE

You are asked to review James Williams, a 76 year old man, post-operatively on the ward. He had a laparotomy and small bowel resection and returned to the ward 2 hours ago. He is receiving intravenous fluids and is on morphine patient-controlled analgesia (PCA). On your arrival, his respiratory rate is 6 breaths per minute and his Glasgow Coma Scale (GCS) score is 7/15.

- What type of assessment approach is appropriate for this situation?
- Suggest the main aim of your assessment at this stage?
- What assessment tools or other measurements might you need to use/obtain for this patient?
- What are the potential causes of this situation?
- What do you think is the main problem in the above-mentioned scenario?

## MEDICAL SCENARIO

John Smith, aged 71, was diagnosed with chronic obstructive pulmonary disease (COPD) 8 years ago following a 10 year history of gradually worsening shortness of breath (SOB) and productive cough in the winter.

Some background information is provided as follows.

- SH:
  - Retired policeman
  - Married with three children and eight grandchildren
  - Lives with wife in three-bedroom house
  - Smoker for 40 years × 10 cigarettes per day = 20 pack-years
- DH:
  - Seretide accuhaler 500 BD
  - Spiriva inhaler 18 µg OD
  - Ventolin inhaler PRN
  - Simvastatin 4 mg OD
- Medical Research Council (MRC) breathlessness score: 4
- Lung function tests:
  - FVC: 3.9 litres (80% predicted)
  - $FEV_1$: 1.2 litres (43% predicted)
  - $FEV_1$/FVC ratio: 31%
- Hospital admission
  - Mr Smith was admitted to hospital via A&E, very anxious, with severe SOB and is currently on a medical ward.
  - His SOB had gradually worsened over the past 7 days with cough producing small amounts of thick yellow sputum and increasing wheeze. He is severely limited by

breathlessness and at present he is in bed and does not feel able to mobilize.
- Observations and arterial blood gases (ABGs) on admission:
  - HR                105 b.p.m.
  - BP                140/90 mmHg
  - temperature       37.8°C
  - $S_pO_2$          89%
  - Oxygen            2 litres via nasal cannula
  - respiratory rate  26 breaths per minute
  - pH                7.36
  - $P_aO_2$          7.2 kPa
  - $P_aCO_2$         7.5 kPa
  - $HCO_3^-$         26.6 mmol l$^{-1}$
  - base excess       +3
- Dyspnoea score at rest = 5 on Borg scale

### Physiotherapy assessment 1 (acute medical)

You are asked to assess this man shortly after his admission to the respiratory ward:

- What type of assessment approach is appropriate for this situation?
- Suggest the main aims of your assessment at this stage
- What assessment tools are you likely to use now?

Mr Smith is initially given amoxicillin 500 mg, ventolin nebulizers 2.5 mg in 2.5 ml QDS and prednisolone tablets 30 mg and improves quickly.

Two days later he is being considered for discharge home.

### Physiotherapy assessment 2 (discharge assessment)

You are asked to re-assess Mr Smith in relation to discharge planning:

- What type of assessment approach is appropriate for this situation?
- What would be the main aim(s) of your assessment at this stage?
- What assessment tools are you likely to use now?

### Physiotherapy assessment 3 (acute community)

Mr Smith is now at home shortly after having been discharged as part of the early discharge support service.

He is sleeping downstairs and has home oxygen at 2 l min⁻¹, which he is using intermittently. His $S_pO_2$ is 90% on air. He is still very breathless at rest and is expectorating thick yellow sputum.

- What type of assessment approach is appropriate for this situation?
- What would be the main aim of your assessment at this stage?
- What assessment tools are you likely to use now?

## Physiotherapy assessment 4 (rehabilitation assessment)

You re-assess Mr Smith 2 weeks later at home during a follow-up visit.

He has recovered from his chest infection and his temperature has now stabilized at 36.8°C. He has stopped using oxygen and his $S_pO_2$ on air is 95%. He is no longer SOBAR (short of breath at rest) but he is still unable to walk far in the house without becoming breathless. He wants to know whether he can go back to sleeping upstairs and whether he can get out. He is very anxious concerning the risk of another attack. He wants to keep using the nebulizers and oxygen 'just in case'.

- What type of assessment approach is appropriate for this situation?
- What would be the main aim of your assessment at this stage?
- What assessment tools are you likely to use now?

## NEUROMUSCULAR SCENARIO

Jack Jones, aged 59, was admitted this afternoon. Over the past week he has been generally unwell, with a temperature and cough. He was diagnosed with motor neurone disease (MND) 18 months ago. Prior to this, he was very fit and active.

- SH
  - He is a former physical education teacher, married with two children. He lives with his wife in a four-bedroom house and has never smoked.
- DH
  - Riluzole
- Lung function tests (last performed 2 months ago) (height 185 cm, weight 86 kg and BMI (body mass index) 25.1)
  - $FEV_1$           2.23 litres (60% predicted)
  - FVC            2.44 litres (52% predicted)
  - $FEV_1$/FVC     91%

- Observations taken on admission (on air):
  - HR          85 b.p.m.
  - BP          120/85 mmHg
  - temperature 37.5°C
  - pH          7.414
  - $P_aCO_2$   7.04 kPa
  - $P_aO_2$    9.27 kPa
  - $HCO_3^-$   30.8 mmol l$^{-1}$
  - $S_aO_2$    93.3%
- What type of assessment approach is appropriate for this situation?
- Suggest the main aims and priorities of your assessment at this stage.
- What type of respiratory disorder does this show?
- Why does an individual with a neuromuscular disorder have respiratory problems?
- What are the implications of this disorder?
- Can you interpret the ABG?
- What assessment tools or other measurements might you need to use/obtain for this patient?

## 4.3 SUGGESTED ANSWERS

Remember these solutions are not all encompassing and you may find it helpful to discuss these scenarios with your supervisor or mentor.

### *SURGICAL SCENARIO (JAMES WILLIAMS)*

- *What type of assessment approach is appropriate for this situation?*
  - In the acute setting a systematic assessment approach is commonly used.
- *Suggest the main aim of your assessment at this stage?*
  - Is the patient safe? Remember: if a patient does not appear well from a handover or when you go to see them, always link with your senior and check: A (airway), B (breathing), C (circulation). They will be able to guide you.
- *What assessment tools or other measurements might you need to use/obtain for this patient?*
  - AVPU or GCS: will be able to tell you how responsive this patient is. Remember: if there has been a change (better or worse), this is important to note and to feed back to the staff on the ward.
  - Pupil response: check whether they are responsive and whether there are any changes; this should also be reported back to the ward team.
  - Pain score: is the patient in pain or is he receiving too much analgesia? If it is the latter, he may not be able to communicate with you.
  - HR and rhythm: does the patient have a pulse? Is it steady? What is the trend? Is HR above BP? Do you need help?
  - BP: does the patient have a stable BP? Is the trend stable? If there is a trend for a falling BP, he may need more fluid or could be bleeding. If you are unsure about the stability of the patient's BP it is important that you ask senior staff for assistance!
  - Re-measure RR: at what rate would you be concerned? What has the trend been – this may tell you if the patient is getting better or worse. Do you need help?
  - Oxygen and saturations: are saturations acceptable and stable? How much oxygen is the patient receiving and is his need for oxygen increasing?
  - Auscultation: are there breath sounds to all zones? Are there any added sounds? If so, where and what may these indicate?

- Palpation: is the chest wall moving or is breathing so shallow that there is little movement and the patient is not effectively ventilating?
- Within 2 hours of surgery there may not be a chest radiograph or any ABGs, but if these have been done they need to be checked.

- *What are the potential causes of this situation?*
  - Neurological problem: if a patient drops their level of consciousness after an operation, it could be due to a neurological incident (e.g. stroke). However, more commonly this is likely to be due to the effects of the anaesthetic or the side-effects of some drugs.
  - Effect of anaesthesia: after an operation (especially prolonged surgical time) patients may remain 'flat' (damped responses) for a period. This may make a patient less responsive and thus lower their GCS. Anaesthetic drugs can also depress the respiratory drive and therefore make a person breathe more slowly and shallowly; however, the patient would be unlikely to be sent to the ward from the recovery area until this was resolved.
  - Effect of analgesia: morphine is a strong analgesic that can depress the respiratory system and cause drowsiness. These effects can happen to a patient postoperatively, especially if they are sensitive to morphine – this can be described as opioid narcosis. In many hospitals, morphine is written up on the drug chart with naloxone – a drug that reverses the effect of morphine. If necessary, ward staff are able to administer this. Signs of opioid narcosis are reduced RR (<8 breaths per minute), reduced level of consciousness and pinpoint pupils.
- *What do you think is the main problem in the above-mentioned scenario?*
  - Too much morphine is the most likely reason for the signs identified in this scenario, but it is important that you fully assess the patient. Although common things are the most likely cause, sometimes it may be the uncommon option that is responsible...a comprehensive assessment ensures that you do not miss anything obvious!

## MEDICAL SCENARIO (JOHN SMITH)
### Physiotherapy assessment 1 (acute medical)
- *What type of assessment approach is appropriate for this situation?*
  - A systematic assessment would be appropriate as this man is in an acute stage of illness.

- *Suggest the main aims of your assessment at this stage.*
  – Once you are satisfied that his airway, breathing and circulation are all adequate and stable, your main focus will be to identify his main problems, i.e. sputum retention, low lung volumes or breathlessness, and then to select physiotherapy management options for treating these problems, if appropriate.
- *What assessment tools might you need to focus on with this man?*
  – Oximetry and ABGs to check that his oxygenation and ventilation remain adequate. Any deterioration should be reported to the medical team.
  – TPR chart is important as he needs frequent monitoring in this acute stage to identify deterioration – look for trends!
  – Respiratory pattern and rate may help to determine whether he would benefit from breathing interventions such as breathing control. These should also be considered alongside ABGs to identify whether he is at risk of respiratory fatigue, which may require non-invasive ventilation.
  – Breathlessness should be discussed and can also be used as an objective marker. It may help to change his position to make this more manageable.
  – Palpation and auscultation will help to identify sputum retention or low lung volumes that might require sputum clearance or positioning.
  – Chest radiograph may be useful in determining any consolidation or collapse to support the above decision.

### Physiotherapy assessment 2 (discharge assessment)

- *What type of assessment approach is appropriate for this situation?*
  – You could include aspects of both systematic and functional assessments in order to determine whether the acute condition that required admission has now stabilized and whether he is likely to need any help to be able to reach his previous level of function.
- *What would be the main aim(s) of your assessment at this stage?*
  – To ensure that he is likely to be able to cope at home and that he understands how to manage his chest clearance and breathlessness, if appropriate. It is also important to explore his mobility and functional ability and make sure he knows how much exercise and activity he can do, and how to monitor and progress this at home.

- *What assessment tools are you likely to use now?*
  - Auscultation and respiratory pattern to check that his chest is clear.
  - Breathlessness: to check that he can use breathing control and can manage his breathlessness, this can also be used as an objective measure and compared with the score on admission.
  - Functional assessment: to ensure that he can manage activities of daily living.
  - Drugs assessment and inhaler technique may be worth checking to find out whether he knows what his medications are for; and what to do if he becomes more breathless or develops sputum retention once at home. Any concerns should be discussed with senior staff prior to discharge.
  - Exercise tolerance/tests: discuss his exercise tolerance and consider carrying out a 6 minute walk test (if appropriate and time allows) to find out how much he can manage in order to advise him regarding exercise at home.

### Physiotherapy assessment 3 (acute community)
- *What type of assessment approach is appropriate for this situation?*
  - A combination of systematic assessment and a functional assessment. Although he is in the community he still appears to have an acute problem; therefore, a systematic assessment approach should not be forgotten.
- *What would be the main aim of your assessment at this stage?*
  - To identify whether he is safe, medically stable and is coping at home.
  - To identify whether there are any problems that require physiotherapy or referral to another service.
  - To ensure that the patient's management has been optimized. In view of the continued breathlessness and sputum production you need to be satisfied that his airway, breathing and circulation are all adequate and are as stable as in the acute setting assessment to ensure that he has not deteriorated.
- *What assessment tools are you likely to use now?*
  - Oxygen delivery assessment: does he still need to use his oxygen? Is he using it for long enough? When does he need to use his oxygen – at rest and/or during activity? Will it be appropriate to consider weaning him off the oxygen? These issues should be discussed with your senior and with medical staff prior to advising the patient.
  - Drug assessment: you need to find out whether he is taking his medication appropriately. Is he taking his inhaler

correctly and using the spacer device? He is still very breathless, so does he require more bronchodilator therapy? Does he need a further course of antibiotics or steroids? Can he be considered for weaning from the nebulizer? (Any concerns regarding medication should be discussed with a senior clinician with authority to prescribe before any decisions are made or any advice is given to the patient.)
- Auscultation and palpation: are there retained secretions and does this support the need for further chest clearance techniques or advice?
- RR and respiratory pattern: is Mr Smith becoming fatigued? How well is he managing his breathlessness?
- Functional assessment: can he manage his activities of daily living? Can he manage to get himself to the bathroom, eat and dress? Is he able to get upstairs or is he too breathless to try at the moment?
- Social assessment: are the services that he requires all available? Does he need any further help to manage at home?

### Physiotherapy assessment 4 (rehabilitation assessment)
- *What type of assessment approach is appropriate for this situation?*
  - A goal-oriented assessment would be most appropriate. (This may lead on to aspects of functional assessment, if required.)
- *What would be the main aim of your assessment at this stage?*
  - To explore his main goals and problems and analyse them further.
  - To help Mr Smith to continue to improve and manage his symptoms.
- *What assessment tools are you likely to use now?*
  - Exercise tests may be appropriate if exercise tolerance is an issue (such as the incremental shuttle walking test or the 6 minute walk test). Does he need to pace himself more effectively when walking? Does he require a walking aid? Is he interested in pulmonary rehabilitation to improve his fitness and, if so, is there a local programme you could refer him to?
  - Breathlessness: would he benefit from further breathing control practice? What is his breathlessness score now? Has it changed from the last review? Does he need advice regarding relaxation and stress?
  - Anxiety regarding a further attack: does he know how to manage another attack and what he should do?

- Drug therapy: does he understand the purpose of the oxygen and nebulizers? Perhaps he needs further education about their use? Is his medication optimal at this point or would he benefit from a further medical review? Would it be appropriate for him to keep antibiotics and steroids at home to use as 'rescue' treatment? (Any decisions regarding medication should be discussed with a senior clinician with authority to prescribe before any advice is given to the patient.)
- Knowledge of disease and self-management: does he know how to manage his COPD on a day-to-day basis? Could he recognize the signs of a chest infection and does he know what to do if he develops another infection?

## NEUROMUSCULAR SCENARIO (JACK JONES)

- *What type of assessment approach is appropriate for this situation?*
  - In the acute setting, a systems-based assessment would be the first choice; however, there are aspects of functional and social assessments that are important to include.
- *Suggest the main aims and priorities of your assessment at this stage.*
  - As ever, the history is key. Motor neurone disease is a progressive degenerative disease characterized by muscle weakness. This affects all muscles, including the respiratory muscles. So, the first part of the assessment needs to be the safety aspect of ensuring that he is maintaining an adequate airway and breathing (ventilation).
- *What type of respiratory disorder does this show?*
  - The ratio between the $FEV_1$/FVC is above normal, and so there is no obstruction to the airflow.
  - The measured volumes for $FEV_1$ and FVC are both down considerably in comparison with the predicted values. Therefore, this is a restrictive lung disorder, due to his weak respiratory muscles.
  - However, this is a progressive disease. The recommendations from the National Institute for Health and Clinical Excellence (NICE) are for spirometry to be repeated every 3 months. These were performed 2 months ago, and so probably do not represent his current respiratory function.
- *Why does an individual with a neuromuscular disorder have respiratory problems?*
  - He has progressive weakness as a result of his disease. This will affect his respiratory muscles over time, and this is reflected in his poor respiratory function.

- *What are the implications of this disorder?*
  - Over time he will find it difficult to breathe in and thus is likely to slip into respiratory failure. This is likely to start at night, and he will not be able to lie flat.
  - The weakness will affect his expiratory muscles, and so airway clearance will become difficult.
  - There is a chance that the weakness will affect his bulbar function and he may well have trouble swallowing. This puts him at risk of aspiration.
- *Can you interpret the ABG?*
  - The pH is normal.
  - $P_aCO_2$ is high.
  - Bicarbonate is high – this compensates for the high $P_aCO_2$.
  - $P_aO_2$ is just below normal range but adequate.
  - This is a compensated respiratory acidosis.
  - In this case, he is not sensitive to oxygen; he is just not maintaining an adequate tidal volume all the time to clear the retained $CO_2$.
- *What assessment tools or other measurements might you need to use/obtain for this patient?*
  - General observation of the patient will tell you a huge amount. Does this patient look distressed and uncomfortable or relaxed? Is the patient talking in complete sentences? If not, this will indicate that he is working hard.
  - Work of breathing: is this patient using his accessory muscles to assist the diaphragm?
  - RR and pattern: will indicate how hard he is working; remember to look at the trend.
  - Breathlessness scoring: formal scoring may not be appropriate in the acute setting. A simple question of 'do you feel breathless?' is probably enough to indicate that he is struggling.
  - Oximetry: will give a quick indication of the oxygenation of the patient.
  - ABGs: will need to be repeated. A rising level of $CO_2$ would indicate a progression in his respiratory failure.
  - Palpation: is his thoracic expansion equal?
  - Auscultation: how much air is being shifted by his respiratory effort and is the air entry equal?
  - Cough assessment: with a progressive weakening of the respiratory muscles, both inspiratory and expiratory, he may not have the ability to cough effectively. Assessment of his ability to clear his own airways is very important. If this is impaired you should consider whether this is a new symptom. It may

be that with an acute infection he now cannot clear his airways, but with treatment he may recover.
- Imaging: in this case a chest radiograph will show the level of expansion of the lungs, and any areas of collapse or consolidation that you may need to treat.
- Lung function tests: there would be some value in repeating these as his disease is progressive. However, this needs to be viewed in the context of the situation. If a patient is in respiratory distress, he or she will not be able to complete the tests.
- Sometimes, end-of-life decisions need to be made in a case like this. This is outside of the remit of this case study but is a subject that could be discussed with a senior clinician.

# Index

Note: Page numbers followed by *b* indicate boxes, *f* indicate figures, and *t* indicate tables.

As the subject of this book is concerned primarily with respiratory assessment, entries under this and "assessment" have been kept to a minimum. Readers are advised to look for more specific terms

Abbreviations used in this index can be found in the "*Normal values*" chapter

*vs.* indicates a comparison or differential diagnosis

## A

ABC assessment, 10*t*
Abdomen, palpation, 142
ABGs *see* Arterial blood gases (ABGs)
Absent breath sounds, 40
Acidosis
   metabolic, 29, 30, 31*t*
   respiratory *see* Respiratory acidosis
Activated prothrombin time (APTT), 50, 52*t*
Actrapid, 90*t*
Acute community patient assessment, 19, 20*t*
   chronic obstructive pulmonary disease, 181–182, 188–189
   functional assessment, 20*t*
Acute respiratory assessments, 9–12, 11*t*
Acute respiratory diseases, arterial blood gases, 32
Adalat, 87*t*
Adenosine, 87*t*
Adrenaline (epinephrine), 87*t*
AEB (atrial ectopic beats), 114*t*
AF *see* Atrial fibrillation (AF)

Aims of assessment, 4–5
Airway protection reflexes, 152
Airway resistance, work of breathing, 177
Alert, AVPU, 43
Alignments, chest X-ray interpretation, 72*t*
Alkalosis
   metabolic, 29, 30, 31*t*
   respiratory *see* Respiratory alkalosis
Ambu bag, 134*f*
Aminoglycosides, 89*t*
Aminophylline, 85*t*
Amiodarone, 87*t*
Amoxicillin, 89*t*
Analgesic drugs, 89*t*
Anti-arrhythmia drugs, 87*t*
Antibiotics, 89*t*
Anticholinergic drugs, 85*t*
Anticoagulant drugs, 90*t*
Anti-epileptic drugs, 90*t*
Antihypertensive drugs, 49, 87*t*
Apical breathing, 155*t*
Apneustic breathing, 155*t*
Apnoea, 155*t*
Arrhythmias, heart rate, 112
Arterial blood gases (ABGs), 25–34
   clinical examples, 32–33
   definition, 25
   documentation, 32
   findings, 26–32, 28*f*, 28*t*
   procedure, 26, 27*f*
   purpose, 26
Arterial pressure, 60
ASB (assisted spontaneous breathing), 174*t*

Aspirin, 90t
Assessment checklists, 9–21
Assisted spontaneous breathing (ASB), 174t
Asthma Quality of Life questionnaire, 149, 150
Ataxic breathing, 155t
Atenolol, 87t
Atracurium, 89t
Atrial ectopic beats (AEB), 114t
Atrial fibrillation (AF), 114t
   ECG, 118f
Atrial flutter (AF), 114t
   ECG, 118f
Atrioventricular block, 114t
Atrovent (ipratropium bromide), 85t
Attachments, 34–36
   definition, 34, 35f
   documentation, 36
   findings, 36
   procedure, 34
   purpose, 34
Auscultation, 36–43
   definition, 36
   documentation, 43
   findings, 37–42
   procedure, 36–37, 38f, 38t
   purpose, 36
Automated blood pressure monitoring, 44f, 45f, 47–48, 47f
AVPU, 43–44
   definition, 43
   documentation, 44
   findings, 44
   procedure, 43
   purpose, 43

## B

Balance assessment, 18
Barrel chest, 75f
Base excess (BE), 28t, 29
BE *see* Base excess (BE)
Beclomethasone, 85t
Bendrofluazide, 87t
Benzylpenicillin, 89t
B$_2$-agonists, 85t
Beta($\beta$)-blockers, 87t
Bicarbonate (HCO$_3^-$), 28t, 29

Blood pressure (BP), 44–49
   automated, 44f, 45f, 47–48, 47f
   definition, 44
   documentation, 49
   findings, 48–49, 169–170
   heart rhythms, 117
   non-invasive, 45–47
   procedure, 45–48
   purpose, 44–45
Blood tests, 49–55, 49t
   documentation, 55
   findings, 50–55
   microbiology, 55
   procedure, 50
   purpose, 50
   *see also specific types*
Body temperature
   findings, 167–169
   normal, 167–169, 169t
   procedure, 167
Bones, chest X-ray, 72t
Borg breathlessness scale, 56
   exercise testing, 103
   findings, 57
   procedure, 56–57, 57t
   purpose, 56
Borg (revised) CR10, 150, 151t
Borg (original) RPE scale, 150, 151t
BP *see* Blood pressure (BP)
Bradycardia, 111–112
   sinus *see* Sinus bradycardia (SB)
Bradypnoea, 157–158
Breathing pattern *see* Respiratory patterns
Breathlessness (dyspnoea) scales, 56–58
   definition, 56
   documentation, 57–58
   findings, 57–58
   procedure, 56–57
   purpose, 56
   *see also specific scales*
Breath sounds, 37–38, 39t
   absent, 40
   bronchial breathing, 39–40, 39t
   coarse crackles, 41, 41t
   crackles, 40–41, 41t
   loud, 40
   normal, 39, 39t
   quiet, 40
   wheezes, 41, 42t

Bronchial breathing, 39–40, 39t
Bronchodilators, 85t
Bruce protocol, treadmill test, 97
Bubbling, chest drains, 66–67
Budesonide, 85t
Bumetanide, 87t

# C

Calcium channel blockers (CCBs), 87t
Capillary refill test, 58–59
Captopril, 87t
Carbamazepine, 90t
Carbocysteine, 85t
Carbon dioxide partial pressure ($P_aCO_2$), 26–27, 28t
Cardiac assessment, chest X-rays, 72t
Cardiac drugs, 87t
Cardiac index, 60
Cardiac markers, 55
Cardiac monitoring (invasive), 59–62
    arterial pressure, 60
    central venous pressure, 61, 62–64, 63f
    continuous thermodilution, 61–62, 61f
    definition, 59–60
    documentation, 62
    findings, 62
    PiCCO, 61–62, 61f
    procedure, 60–62
    pulmonary artery catheter (Swan–Ganz), 61, 62
    purpose, 60
Cardiopulmonary exercise test (CPET), 97, 98f
Cardiovascular system (CVS)
    acute respiratory assessment, 11t
    general surgery patient assessment, 13t
    intensive therapy unit assessment, 14t
    medical patient assessment, 15t
Case histories, 179–192
    chronic obstructive pulmonary disease, 3b, 180
    medical scenario, 180–182, 186–190
    neuromuscular assessment, 182–183, 190–192
    surgery, 179–180, 185–186

CCBs (calcium channel blockers), 87t
Cefaclor, 89t
Cefetaxime, 89t
Central nervous system (CNS)
    acute respiratory assessment, 11t
    general surgery patient assessment, 13t
    intensive therapy unit assessment, 14t
Central venous pressure (CVP), 61, 62–64, 63f
Cephalosporins, 89t
Cerebral perfusion pressure (CPP), 64–65
Checklists, 9–21
Chest drains, 65–68
    definition, 65, 66f
    documentation, 68
    findings, 66–68
    procedure, 65, 67f
    purpose, 65
Chest imaging, 68–74
    definition, 68
    documentation, 74
    findings, 70–71
    procedure, 69
    purpose, 68–69
    *see also specific methods*
Chest wall shape, 74–76
    definition, 74
    documentation, 76
    findings, 74–76, 75f
    procedure, 74
    purpose, 74
Chest wall, work of breathing, 176
Chest X-rays (CXR), 68–69
    interpretation, 70f, 72f, 70–73, 72t
    review questions, 71t
Cheyne–Stokes respiration, 155t
Chronic cough, 79–80
Chronic obstructive pulmonary disease (COPD)
    acute community patient assessment, 181–182, 188–189
    case histories, 180
    case history, 3b
    discharge assessment, 181, 187–188
    physiotherapy assessment, 181–182, 186–190
    rehabilitation assessment, 182, 189–190

Chronic Respiratory Disease Questionnaire (CRQ), 149
Chronic respiratory diseases
  arterial blood gases, 32
  cyanosis, 81
Ciclosporin, 90$t$
Classification of respiratory problems, 8
Clexane, 90$t$
Clinical reasoning, 7–8
Clubbing *see* Digital clubbing
CMV (continuous mandatory ventilation), 173–174, 174$t$
CNS *see* Central nervous system (CNS)
Coagulation screen, 50, 52$t$
  *see also specific screens*
Coarse crackles, 41, 41$t$
Codeine, 89$t$
Cognitive assessment, 16$t$
Colour, sputum assessment, 162
Commercial monitors, heart rate, 111
Community, assessment in, 5–6
  hospital admissions, 6, 7$f$
  re-evaluation, 6
Compensation, 29–31, 30$b$, 31$t$
Computer tomography (CT), 69
Consent, 78–79
Constant speed exercise tests, 99
Continuous mandatory ventilation (CMV), 173–174, 174$t$
Continuous positive airways pressure (CPAP), 174$t$
Continuous thermodilution, 61–62, 61$f$
Coordination assessment, 18
COPD *see* Chronic obstructive pulmonary disease (COPD)
Cough assessment, 79–81
CPAP (continuous positive airways pressure), 174$t$
CPET (cardiopulmonary exercise test), 97, 98$f$
CPP (cerebral perfusion pressure), 64–65
Crackles, 40–41, 41$t$
C-reactive protein (CRP), 50, 52$t$
Creatinine, 53$t$
Critical care *see* Intensive therapy units (critical care)
CRP (C-reactive protein), 50, 52$t$

CRQ (Chronic Respiratory Disease Questionnaire), 149
CT (computer tomography), 69
Cuff size, sphygmomanometer, 46$t$
CVP (central venous pressure), 61, 62–64, 63$f$
CVS *see* Cardiovascular system (CVS)
CXR *see* Chest X-rays (CXR)
Cyanosis, 81–82

# D

Database
  general assessments, 10$t$
  general surgery patient assessment, 13$t$
  intensive therapy unit assessment, 14$t$
  medical patient assessment, 15$t$
Dead space, 171
Deep tendon reflexes, 152, 153
Dehydration, 107
Dermatomes, 82–84
  definition, 82, 82$f$
  documentation, 82$f$, 83
  findings, 83
  procedure, 83
  purpose, 83
Dexamethasone, 90$t$
Diabetes mellitus, exercise testing, 101
Diamorphine, 89$t$
Diaphragmatic breathing, 155$t$
Diaphragm, chest X-ray, 72$t$
Diffusion, lung function tests, 126
Digital clubbing, 77, 78$f$
  causes, 77$t$
Digoxin, 87$t$
Diltiazem, 87$t$
Discharge assessments, chronic obstructive pulmonary disease, 181, 187–188
Diuretics, 87$t$
DNAR (do not attempt resuscitation), 158
DNAse (Dornase Alfa), 85$t$
Dobutamine, 87$t$
Documentation
  attachments, 36
  auscultation, 43

Documentation *(Continued)*
 AVPU, 44
 blood pressure, 49
 blood tests, 55
 breathlessness (dyspnoea) scales, 57–58
 cardiac monitoring (invasive), 62
 chest drains, 68
 chest imaging, 74
 chest wall shape, 76
 consent, 78–79
 cough assessment, 80
 dermatomes, 82*f*, 83
 drugs (medication), 91
 early warning scores, 93
 end-tidal carbon dioxide, 97
 exercise testing, 103
 fluid balance, 106*f*, 107–108
 Glasgow Coma Scale, 110
 heart rate, 112
 heart rhythms, 119
 intracranial pressure, 122
 level of consciousness, 123
 lung function tests, 128
 muscle charting (Oxford grading), 131
 oxygen delivery, 139
 pain scores, 140
 palpation, 143
 percussion note, 144
 pulse oximetry, 146
 pupils, 148
 rating of perceived exertion, 151
 reflexes, 153
 respiratory patterns, 154
 respiratory rate, 158
 resuscitation status, 160
 sputum assessment, 163
 swallow assessment, 165
 TPR (temperature, pulse and respiration) chart, 170
 ventilation–perfusion matching, 172
 ventilators, 174–175
Do not attempt resuscitation (DNAR), 158
Dopamine, 87*t*
Dornase Alfa (DNAse), 85*t*
Doxycycline, 89*t*
Draining, chest drains, 67
Drugs (medications), 84–91, 85*t*, 87*t*, 89*t*, 90*t*

Drugs (medications) *(Continued)*
 definition, 84
 documentation, 91
 findings, 84–91
 procedure, 84
 purpose, 84
 *see also specific drugs*
Dull sound, percussion, 144
Dyspnoea scales *see* Breathlessness (dyspnoea) scales

# E

Early warning scores (EWSs), 91–93, 92*t*
Ear thermometer, 168*f*
ECGs (electrocardiograms), 113, 117*f*, 118*f*, 119*f*
Effectiveness, cough, 79
Efficacy, ventilators, 173
Electrocardiograms (ECGs), 113, 117*f*, 118*f*, 119*f*
Electronic thermometers, 167
Enalapril, 87*t*
End-tidal carbon dioxide (ET$co_2$), 93–97, 94*f*
 definition, 93–94
 documentation, 97
 findings, 96
 normal values, 96
 procedure, 95
 purpose, 95
 ventilation, 96
Environment, exercise testing, 101
Epinephrine (adrenaline), 87*t*
Erythrocyte cell count, 51*t*
ET$co_2$ *see* End-tidal carbon dioxide (ET$co_2$)
EWSs (early warning scores), 91–93, 92*t*
Exercise testing, 97–103
 after test, 102
 definition, 97
 documentation, 103
 findings, 103
 preceding concerns, 99–101
 pre-test measurements, 102
 procedure, 97–102
 purpose, 97
 during testing, 102
 *see also specific tests*

Exercise tolerance, 103–105
  documentation, 105
Expansion, chest X-ray, 72*t*
Expiratory reserve volume, 124*t*
Externally paced exercise tests, 98, 99*f*
Extrathoracic structures, chest X-ray, 72*t*
Eyes (E), Glasgow Coma Scale, 109

## F

Face mask, oxygen delivery, 134, 134*f*, 138*t*
FBC (full blood count), 50, 51*t*
Fentanyl, 89*t*
FEV$_1$ *see* Forced expiratory volume in the first second (FEV$_1$)
Fever (pyrexia), 169
Fibrinogen levels, 52*t*
Field exercise tests, 98–99
  constant speed, 99
  externally paced, 98, 99*f*
  incremental speed, 99
  maximal, 99
  self-paced, 98
  submaximal, 99
Fields, chest X-ray, 72*t*
Fixed performance devices, oxygen delivery, 134, 137*t*
Flow–volume loop curve
  definition, 125*t*
  lung problems, 128
Flucloxacillin, 89*t*
Fluid balance, 105–108
  documentation, 106*f*, 107–108
Fluid loss, 107
Fluid overload, 107
Fluticasone, 85*t*
Forced expiratory volume in the first second (FEV$_1$)
  definition, 124, 125*t*
  normal, 127
Forced vital capacity (FVC)
  definition, 124, 125*t*
  normal, 127
Formeterol, 85*t*
Frusemide, 87*t*
Full blood count (FBC), 50, 51*t*
Functional assessment, 5, 17–19
  acute community patient assessment, 20*t*
  balance/coordination, 18

Functional assessment *(Continued)*
  functional mobility, 18–19, 18*t*
  muscle strength, 18, 18*t*
  range of movement, 17, 17*t*
  sensation, 18
Functional mobility assessment, 18–19, 18*t*
Functional residual capacity, 124*t*
Funnel chest (pes excavatum), 74, 75*f*
Furosemide, 87*t*
FVC *see* Forced vital capacity (FVC)

## G

Gadgets, chest X-ray interpretation, 72*t*
GCS *see* Glasgow Coma Scale (GCS)
General assessments, 9, 10*t*
General observations, 10*t*
General surgery patient assessment, 12–13, 13*t*
Gentamicin, 89*t*
Glasgow Coma Scale (GCS), 108–110, 108*t*
  normal score, 109
Gliclazide, 90*t*
Global ejection fraction, 60
Glucose, 55, 55*t*
Glyceryl trinitrate (GTN), 87*t*
Goal-oriented assessment, 5, 6*f*, 16–17, 16*t*
GTN (glyceryl trinitrate), 87*t*

## H

Haematocrit, 51*t*
Haemoglobin levels, 51*t*
HCO$_3^-$ *see* Bicarbonate (HCO$_3^-$)
Head box, oxygen delivery, 134
Heart block, 114*t*
  ECG, 119*f*
Heart rate (HR), 110–112
  arrhythmias, 112
  exercise testing, 103
  manual pulse, 110
  *see also* Pulse
Heart rhythms, 112–119, 114*t*
  blood pressure, 117
Heparin, 90*t*
Hospital admissions, community-based assessment, 6, 7*f*

HR *see* Heart rate (HR)
Humidification, oxygen delivery, 138
Humulin, 90*t*
Hydrocortisone, 90*t*
Hypercapnia, 26–27
　carbon dioxide partial pressure, 26
Hyperinflation, localized, 155*t*
Hyperlactinaemia, 52–53
Hyperpyrexia, 169
Hypertension, 48
Hypertonic saline, 85*t*
Hyperventilation, 155*t*
Hypocapnia, 27
　carbon dioxide partial pressure, 26
Hypopnoea, 155*t*
Hypotension, 48
Hypothermia, 169
Hypoventilation, 155*t*
Hypoxaemia, oxygenation, 31

## I

Ibuprofen, 89*t*
Immunosuppressant drugs, 90*t*
Incremental speed exercise tests, 99
Inotropes, 49, 87*t*
INR (international normalized ratio), prothrombin time, 50, 52*t*
Inspiratory reserve volume, 124*t*
Insulins, 90*t*
Intensive care unit (ITU, critical care) charts, 122–123, 122*f*
Intensive therapy units (critical care), 1, 2*f*, 3*f*
　assessment, 13–15, 14*t*
International normalized ratio (INR), prothrombin time, 50, 52*t*
Interpretation, chest X-rays, 70*f*, 72*f*, 70–73, 72*t*
Intracranial pressure (ICP), 120–122, 121*f*
　normal values, 120
　raised, 120–121
　treatment effects, 121
Invasive cardiac monitoring *see* Cardiac monitoring (invasive)
Ipratropium bromide (Atrovent), 85*t*
ITU *see* Intensive therapy units (critical care)

## K

K⁺ (potassium), 54–55, 54*t*
Knee-jerk (patella) reflex, 152
Kussmaul's respiration, 155*t*
Kyphosis, 76

## L

Labetalol, 87*t*
Lactate levels, 52–53, 52*t*
Lactic acidosis, 52–53
Level of consciousness, 123
　*see also* AVPU; Glasgow Coma Scale (GCS)
LFTs *see* Lung function tests (LFTs)
Lidoflaxine, 87*t*
Listening, work of breathing, 176
Load, work of breathing, 176
Localized hyperinflation, 155*t*
Loud breath sounds, 40
Lower chest breathing, 155*t*
Lower limbs, palpation, 142–143
Lung compliance, work of breathing, 177
Lung function tests (LFTs), 124–129
　combined problems, 128
　definition, 124–125, 124*t*
　documentation, 128
　findings, 124*t*, 126–128, 127*f*
　interpretation, 127–128
　obstructive problems, 127, 128*f*
　procedure, 126
　purpose, 125–126
　restrictive problems, 128, 128*f*
　*see also specific lung function measurements*
Lung volumes, 124–129

## M

Magnetic resonance imaging (MRI), 69
Management, assessment in, 1
Manual pulse
　heart rate, 110
　sites, 111*t*
MAP (mean arterial pressure), 60
Maximal exercise tests, 99
MCV (mean corpuscular volume), 51*t*
Mean arterial pressure (MAP), 60

Mean corpuscular volume (MCV), 51*t*
Medical patient assessment, 15, 15*t*
Medical Research Council (MRC) breathlessness scale, 56
  findings, 58
  procedure, 57, 58*t*
  purpose, 56
Medical scenario, case histories, 180–182, 186–190
Medical stability, acute community patient assessment, 20*t*
Medication *see* Drugs (medications)
Metabolic acidosis, 29, 30, 31*t*
Metabolic alkalosis, 29, 30, 31*t*
Microbiology, blood tests, 55
Midazolam, 89*t*
Mixtard, 90*t*
Morphine, 89*t*
Motor (M), Glasgow Coma Scale, 109
MRC breathlessness scale *see* Medical Research Council (MRC) breathlessness scale
MRI (magnetic resonance imaging), 69
MS *see* Musculoskeletal system (MS)
Mucolytics, 85*t*
Muscle charting (Oxford grading), 128*f*, 129–131
Muscle strength, functional assessment, 18, 18*t*
Musculoskeletal system (MS)
  acute respiratory assessment, 11*t*
  general surgery patient assessment, 13*t*
  goal-oriented assessment, 16*t*
  intensive therapy unit assessment, 14*t*
Myotomes, 131–133, 132*f*

## N

Na+ (sodium), 54, 54*t*
Nasal cannula, oxygen delivery, 134, 134*f*, 138*t*
Neurological system
  goal-oriented assessment, 16*t*
  reflexes, 152
  *see also* Central nervous system (CNS)
Neuromuscular assessment, case histories, 182–183, 190–192
Nifedipine, 87*t*
NIV (non-invasive ventilation), 174*t*
Non-invasive blood pressure monitoring, 45–47
Non-invasive ventilation (NIV), 174*t*
Non-rebreathe mask, oxygen delivery, 138*t*
Non-steroidal anti-inflammatory drugs (NSAIDs), 89*t*
Noradrenaline (norepinephrine), 87*t*
Norepinephrine (noradrenaline), 87*t*
  body temperature, 167–169, 169*t*
  end-tidal carbon dioxide ($ETco_2$), 96
  forced expiratory volume in the first second ($FEV_1$), 127
  forced vital capacity (FVC), 127
  Glasgow Coma Scale, 109
  intracranial pressure, 120
  pupils, 148
  respiratory rate (RR), 157
  $S_po_2$ (pulse oximetry), 146
  ventilation–perfusion matching, 171–172
Not for resuscitation (NFR), 158
NSAIDs (non-steroidal anti-inflammatory drugs), 89*t*
Nuclear medicine, chest imaging, 69

## O

Obstructive problems
  chest wall shape, 76
  lung function tests, 127, 128*f*
Opiate drugs, 89*t*
Oxford grading (muscle charting), 128*f*, 129–131
Oxygen, 85*t*
Oxygenation, arterial blood gases, 31
Oxygen delivery, 133–139
  definition, 133
  documentation, 139
  findings, 138–139
  fixed performance devices, 134, 137*t*
  humidification, 138
  methods, 133–134, 134*f*
  procedure, 133–138
  purpose, 133
  variable flow devices, 138, 138*t*

Oxygen partial pressure ($P_aO_2$), 28t
Oxygen saturation ($S_aO_2$), 28t

## P

$P_aCO_2$ see Carbon dioxide partial pressure ($P_aCO_2$)
PACS (picture archiving and communication system), 69
Pain
  AVPU, 43
  chest drains, 67–68
  palpation, 142
Pain scores, 139–140, 140t
Palpation, 140–143
  definition, 140
  documentation, 143
  findings, 142–143
  procedure, 141, 141f
  purpose, 140–141
  work of breathing, 176
Pancuronium, 89t
$P_aO_2$ see Oxygen partial pressure ($P_aO_2$)
Paracetamol, 89t
Paradoxical movements, palpation, 142
Paralysing agents, 89t
Partial pressure of carbon dioxide see Carbon dioxide partial pressure ($P_aCO_2$)
Partial pressure of oxygen see Oxygen partial pressure ($P_aO_2$)
Patella (knee-jerk) reflex, 152
Peak cough flow, 80
Peak expiratory flow rate (PEFR)
  definition, 124, 125t
  procedure, 126
PEEP (positive end-expiratory pressure), 174t
PEFR see Peak expiratory flow rate (PEFR)
Penicillins, 89t
Percussion note, 143–144, 144f
Perfusion, lung function tests, 126
Pes carinatum (pigeon chest), 74, 75f
Pes excavatum (funnel chest), 74, 75f
PFSDQ (Pulmonary Functional Status and Dyspnoea questionnaire), 149
pH, 26, 28t
Phenytoin, 90t
Phyllocontin, 85t
Physiotherapy assessment, chronic obstructive pulmonary disease, 181–182, 186–190
Physiotherapy problems, intensive therapy unit assessment, 14–15
PiCCO, 61–62, 61f
Picture archiving and communication system (PACS), 69
Pigeon chest (pes carinatum), 74, 75f
Plantar reflex, 153
Plastic strip thermometers, 167
Platelet count, 51t
Pleural rubs, 42, 42t
Positive end-expiratory pressure (PEEP), 174t
Postural hypotension, 48
Potassium ($K^+$), 54–55, 54t
Prednisolone, 90t
Pressure support (PS), 173–174, 174t
Propofol, 89t
Prothrombin time (PT), 50, 52t
PS (pressure support), 173–174, 174t
Psychological assessment, 16t
PT (prothrombin time), 50, 52t
Pulmonary artery catheter (Swan–Ganz), 61, 62
Pulmonary Functional Status and Dyspnoea questionnaire (PFSDQ), 149
Pulmonary function tests see Lung function tests (LFTs)
Pulse
  findings, 169–170
  procedure, 167
Pulse oximetry, 145–146, 145f
Pupil reflex, 152, 153
Pupils, 147–148, 147f
  normal values, 148
  see also Glasgow Coma Scale (GCS)
Pursed lip breathing, 155t
Pyrexia (fever), 169

## Q

Quality of life questionnaires, 148–150
  *see also* specific questionnaires
Quiet breath sounds, 40

## R

Radiography *see* Chest X-rays (CXR)
Raised intracranial pressure, 120–121
Ramsay sedation score, 161*t*
Range of movement, functional assessment, 17, 17*t*
Rating of perceived exertion (RPE), 150–152, 151*t*
Reasons for assessment, 4
Red blood cell count, 51*t*
Re-evaluation, community-based assessment, 6
Reflexes, 152–153
  *see also* specific reflexes
Rehabilitation assessment, 12, 20*t*
  chronic obstructive pulmonary disease, 182, 189–190
Renal system
  acute respiratory assessment, 11*t*
  general surgery patient assessment, 13*t*
  intensive therapy unit assessment, 14*t*
Residual volume, 124*t*
Resonant percussion note, 144
Respiration
  palpation, 142
  procedure, 167
Respiratory acidosis, 29, 31*t*
  carbon dioxide partial pressure ($P_aCO_2$), 26
Respiratory alkalosis, 29, 31*t*
  carbon dioxide partial pressure ($P_aCO_2$), 26
Respiratory diseases
  acute, arterial blood gases, 32
  chronic *see* Chronic respiratory diseases
Respiratory failure, arterial blood gases, 31–32
Respiratory muscle strength, 176
Respiratory patterns, 153–154
  definitions, 155*t*
  work of breathing, 176
  *see also* specific patterns

*Respiratory Physiotherapy: An On-Call Survival Guide*, 8
Respiratory rate (RR), 156–158
  bradypnoea, 157–158
  findings, 169–170
  normal range, 157
  tachypnoea, 157
  work of breathing, 176
Respiratory system
  acute respiratory assessment, 11*t*
  general surgery patient assessment, 13*t*
  goal-oriented assessment, 16*t*
  intensive therapy unit assessment, 14*t*
  medical patient assessment, 15*t*
Restrictive problems
  chest wall shape, 74–76
  lung function tests, 128, 128*f*
Resuscitation bag, 134
Resuscitation forms, 159, 159*f*
Resuscitation status, 158–160
Review questions, chest X-rays, 71*t*
Riker Sedation-Agitation Scale, 161*t*
RPE (rating of perceived exertion), 150–152, 151*t*
RR *see* Respiratory rate (RR)

## S

Salbutamol, 85*t*
Salmeterol, 85*t*
$S_aO_2$ *see* Oxygen saturation ($S_aO_2$)
Saturation of oxygen *see* Oxygen saturation ($S_aO_2$)
SB *see* Sinus bradycardia (SB)
Scoliosis, 76
Sedation/agitation score, 160–161, 161*t*
Sedative drugs, 89*t*
Self-paced exercise tests, 98
Sensation, functional assessment, 18
SGRQ-C (St Georges Respiratory Questionnaire for COPD), 149
Shallow breathing, 155*t*
Short Form 36 (SF 36), 149, 150
Short Form Chronic Respiratory Disease Questionnaire (SF CRQ), 149

Shunts, 171
Shuttle walking test, 99*f*
SIMV (synchronized intermittent ventilation), 173–174, 174*t*
Sinus bradycardia (SB), 114*t*
   ECG, 117*f*
Sinus rhythms (SR), 114*t*
   ECG, 117*f*
Sinus tachycardia (ST), 114*t*
   ECG, 117*f*
Sites, manual pulse, 111*t*
Smell, sputum assessment, 163
Social assessment
   acute community patient assessment, 20*t*
   goal-oriented assessment, 16*t*
Sodium ($Na^+$), 54, 54*t*
Solid feel, percussion note, 144
Sphygmomanometer, 44, 45–47
   cuff size, 46*t*
Spirometry, 126
Spironolactone, 87*t*
$S_pO_2$ (pulse oximetry), 145–146
   normal values, 146
Sputum assessment, 161–163
   colour, 162
   smell, 163
   taste, 163
   viscosity, 163
   volume, 162
SR *see* Sinus rhythms (SR)
ST *see* Sinus tachycardia (ST)
Steroids, 85*t*, 90*t*
Stethoscope, 36, 37*f*
St Georges Respiratory Questionnaire for COPD (SGRQ-C), 149
Stridor, 42, 42*t*
Stroke volume index, 59
Subjective questions, general assessments, 10*t*
Submaximal exercise tests, 99
Suppression, cough, 79
Supraventricular tachycardia (SVT), 114*t*
   ECG, 118*f*
Surgery, case histories, 179–180, 185–186
Surgical emphysema, palpation, 142
Surgical incisions, 163–164
   sites, 164*f*
SVT *see* Supraventricular tachycardia (SVT)
Swallow assessment, 164–165
Swan–Ganz catheter, 61, 62
Swinging, chest drains, 66
Synchronized intermittent ventilation (SIMV), 173–174, 174*t*
Systemic vascular resistance, 60
Systems-based assessment, 5

## T

Tachycardia
   heart rate, 111
   sinus *see* Sinus tachycardia (ST)
   supraventricular *see* Supraventricular tachycardia (SVT)
   ventricular *see* Ventricular tachycardia (VT)
Tachypnoea, 157
Taste, sputum assessment, 163
Technology, intensive therapy unit assessment, 14
Temperature *see* Body temperature
Tender loving care (TLC), 158
Terbutaline, 85*t*
Tetracyclines, 89*t*
Theophylline, 85*t*
Thermometers, electronic, 167
Thermometer, tympanic (ear), 168*f*
Thoracic kyphoscoliosis, 75*f*
Thoracoplasty, 76
Thorax, palpation, 142
Three-lead ECGs, 113
Tiotropium, 85*t*
TLC (tender loving care), 158
Total lung capacity, 124*t*
TPR (temperature, pulse and respiration) chart, 165–170, 166*f*
Tracheostomy mask, 134, 134*f*
Treadmill test, Bruce protocol, 97
Twelve-lead ECGs, 113
Tympanic (ear) thermometer, 168*f*

## U

U&Es (urea and electrolytes), 53, 53*t*
Ultrasound imaging, 69
Unresponsive, AVPU, 43
Upper limbs, palpation, 142–143
Urea and electrolytes (U&Es), 53, 53*t*
Urine output, 105–108

## V

Valproate, 90t
Variable flow devices, oxygen delivery, 138, 138t
Vasodilators, 87t
VEB (ventricular ectopic beat), 114t
Vecuronium, 89t
Ventilation, lung function tests, 126
Ventilation–perfusion (V/Q) matching, 170–172
 normal lungs (adults), 171–172
 terminology, 171
Ventilators, 172–175
 documentation, 174–175
 efficacy, 173
 model of, 173
 modes, 173–174
  *see also specific modes*
 oxygen delivery, 134, 134f
 terminology, 173, 174t
 ventilation–perfusion matching, 172
Ventricular ectopic beat (VEB), 114t
Ventricular fibrillation (VF), 114t
 ECG, 119f
Ventricular tachycardia (VT), 114t
 ECG, 118f
Verapamil, 87t
Verbal (V), Glasgow Coma Scale, 109
VF *see* Ventricular fibrillation (VF)
Vibrant feel, percussion note, 144
Viscosity, sputum assessment, 163
Vital capacity, 124t
Vital signs chart *see* TPR (temperature, pulse and respiration) chart
$VO_2$, exercise testing, 103
Voice, AVPU, 43
Voltarol, 89t
Volume, sputum assessment, 162
V/Q matching *see* Ventilation–perfusion (V/Q) matching
VT *see* Ventricular tachycardia (VT)

## W

Warfarin, 90t
WBC (white blood cell count), 51t
Wheezes, 41, 42t
White blood cell count (WBC), 51t
Work of breathing, 175–177

## X

Xanthines, 85t